MIND
OVER
SCATTER

CONQUER ANY TEST WITH
SHARPER FOCUS AND LESS STRESS

NIROSHA RUWAN, JD, IMTA CMT-P

Free Audio

READ THIS FIRST

To help you get the best experience with this book, I would like to give you the audio recordings of mindfulness practices taught in this book. I've found readers who download and use these audio recordings are able to implement and get results faster.

To Download Go To:

www.MindOverScatterBook.com/audio

Dedicated to my daughters,
Shiyana and Ashani,
who inspire me every day

This book is for informational purposes only. It does not replace the advice of a health care professional. The names and details of individuals have been changed in order to protect their privacy. The author and publisher disclaim all liability arising from the use of any information contained in this book.

ISBN (Paperback) 978-1-7362454-1-5
ISBN (ebook) 978-1-7362454-0-8

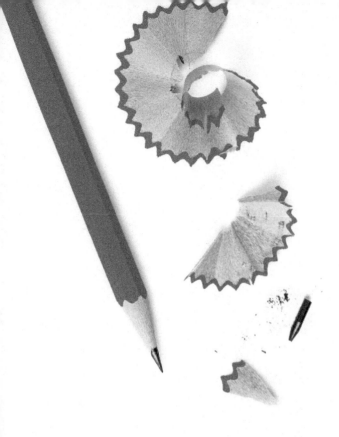

CONTENTS

INTRODUCTION

Does your life sometimes seem to be a never-ending series of tests? Midterms, final exams, and those dreaded standardized tests where you are convinced your entire future depends on the outcome? You know you *should* be preparing for the tests, but you avoid the task as much as possible or simply don't have the time to study. Chances are you're drowning in homework and other commitments such as sports, extracurriculars, volunteer work, and all the other things you've been told you should be doing to build up your résumé.

> "It seems like you're in a constant pressure cooker seasoned with unrealistic expectations, and it's stressful."

Add to that the stresses of a *worldwide pandemic* and its aftermath. You may be grappling with campus closures, illness, canceled events, and distance learning, and all the associated anxiety, economic hardship, and uncertainty that comes with this unprecedented time. Yeah, you have to deal with that, too.

It seems like you're in a constant pressure cooker seasoned with unrealistic expectations, and it's stressful. In the midst of all this, having an upcoming Very Important Test can loom over your life like a heavy, dark cloud.

You may be full of anxiety about upcoming tests and alternating between freaking out and procrastinating. Even if you're one of those lucky students who don't get any test-day jitters, you may still feel consumed with the pressure to excel.

But what can you do? You know you have to take the tests, and you know you want to do well.

You know your test scores will help determine your GPA and your chances of admissions, whether you are applying for college or graduate school. High test scores can also help you land internships and jobs.

Maybe you grit your teeth, grimace, and somehow push through. You may sacrifice your health, and you may not reach your full potential, but you'll just keep grinding away, doing what most students do to prepare for tests: treating it as a painful, uncomfortable rite of passage that you somehow need to get through.

This Book Provides an Alternative

What if you found a way to actually enjoy preparing for and taking tests — and could perform better on them? What if you could become more focused and free up some of your time? Imagine feeling calmer and less stressed while your test scores keep increasing. Sounds impossible, right?

It's not a magic pill; it's a practice called mindfulness. And it really works.

Mindfulness helps your mind stay focused on a task and stay in the present moment. As you study for and take the test, mindfulness can help improve your cognitive abilities. You can learn mindfulness through meditation and other practices, and this book provides a specific road map of how to use mindfulness to improve test performance.

Researchers have found that mindfulness is associated with better academic performance and higher test scores.

What's more, the research has also shown that mindfulness decreases stress and can make you happier too.[1] Not a bad side effect.

While this book is primarily directed to students in high school and college, it can help anyone who wants to score higher on tests with less stress. It can also be used by parents, teachers, and counselors to guide and support students.

How Mindfulness Helped Me

One year, while I was a college student at Harvard, my wrists stopped working. I couldn't type. I couldn't even carry my dining hall tray. Doctors couldn't diagnose me, and splints and physical therapy didn't help me. It was right before final exams and an onslaught of deadlines for papers. It was as though I had been stopped in my tracks while I was running full speed ahead. I was devastated.

The physical pain was so severe, I knew it couldn't be all in my head. But it turned out that even though the pain and immobility were real, it was stress that had shut down my body.

Meditation became a tool that helped me with my recovery, allowing me to confront emotions I simply didn't think I had time to deal with before.

In the high-pressure environment of Harvard, it's not surprising that I felt there was no time to pause. Just like many of my classmates, I kept churning out work to meet deadlines, reaching goals, and immediately making new ones. I let concerns about my health fall to the wayside. I know many students today feel the same pressure, no matter what grade or school they are in.

[1] Madhav Goyal et al., "Meditation Programs for Psychological Stress and Well-being: A Systematic Review and Meta-analysis," *JAMA Internal Medicine* 174, no.3 (2014): 357–58, https://doi.org/10.1001/jamainternmed.2013.13018.

While I initially turned to meditation to help address stress, I found that the practice actually helped my performance as a student, especially during final exams and tests. It allowed me to focus better — and for longer periods of time — and I felt more at ease while engaging in difficult analytical tasks. Along with my health, my academic performance also improved.

Through that experience, I learned that the goals of decreasing stress and improving grades and test scores are actually complementary. There is a way to engage in self-care that will also make you a better student. It's not a zero-sum game.

"Mindfulness can boost academic performance while reducing stress, and also provide a host of other benefits."

The academic stress in my life didn't ease up. I decided to apply to law school, which meant I had to take the LSAT. Once I was in law school, I was confronted with even more papers and exams, not to mention the incessant pressure to score well. Meditation offered me a way to consistently relax and release tension so it didn't build up internally like I was in a pressure cooker.

Mindfulness meditation helped me so much as a student and beyond that I felt inspired to learn more about it and share this practice with others. I completed the training in mindfulness facilitation at the Mindfulness Awareness Research Center at UCLA, where I studied with faculty who had firsthand experience with the clinical research on mindfulness. I also gained familiarity with specific mindfulness courses that were used by researchers in studies about the benefits of mindfulness.

I found that scientific research actually supports what I had discovered from my own experience — that mindfulness can boost academic performance while reducing stress, and also provide a host of other benefits.

I now regularly teach research-based mindfulness to students grappling with the demands of school and daily life. Many students tell me that learning mindfulness has been "life changing," or "the best thing I've ever done."

I'm eager to share these practices with you, and I'm confident that you, too, can reap benefits.

If you're reading this book, you likely care about your grades and test scores. You're probably driven and motivated to do well. It's my sincere hope that this book can help you approach your test-taking with calm and ease and address stress before it overwhelms you.

Is Mindfulness Guaranteed to Work?

Learning mindfulness doesn't guarantee you'll get a perfect score on your tests, but the research and scientific studies on mindfulness show that practicing mindfulness in a particular way is likely to boost your performance. There's also a good chance you'll experience benefits in your life outside of test performance. Finding the time to pause, take a breath, and find stillness is more important than ever in the frantic, fast-paced world of high-stakes academics.

As I mentioned, mindfulness is not a magic pill you can take to increase your test scores. You need to put in some effort to learn the basic practices and implement the steps described in this book. Ultimately, it's up to you to follow the instructions and practice — no one can do it for you. But giving it a go with the help of a guide is a lot easier than trying it on your own.

The real question is whether you're tired of the stress, pressure, and ineffectiveness of your current methods of test-taking and if you're ready to try something new? And even if you aren't currently dissatisfied or overwhelmed with test-taking, are you eager to try research-proven methods of studying more efficiently, improving your performance, and becoming happier?

The Growing Popularity of Mindfulness

If mindfulness is such an amazing tool, why isn't everyone doing it? Indeed, in recent years, there has been a steadily increasing popularity of mindfulness in many fields, including health and the law. Mindfulness is being taught in education settings and integrated into workplaces. It's especially popular among tech companies such as Google, which offers extensive mindfulness training for its employees. Mindfulness is also prescribed by doctors and mental health professionals and often cited as an important component of wellness.

As awareness of mindfulness has grown, it has been featured on the cover of Time Magazine and even championed by members of Congress.

How Is This Book Different from Other Mindfulness Guides or Meditation Apps?

Sure, there's a lot of information out there on the general topics of mindfulness and meditation, but this book is unique because it provides a step-by-step guide on how to use mindfulness for the specific purpose of improving test performance.

Many different teachers, websites, books, and apps offer information on the overall subject. It can be confusing to know who to believe, what practice to try or where to start. There are many popular apps with guided meditations and meditation timers available. These can be great for you to learn and practice the fundamentals, but none of them will focus on the topic at hand and take the guesswork out of mindfulness.

For this book, I've reviewed clinical research studies on mindfulness, and I'm familiar with the specific practices used by researchers when they have concluded that mindfulness can be helpful for academic performance. In the popular press, the word mindfulness is often used loosely, but in academic research, mindfulness is usually associated with a specific training curriculum and practice regimen. While the specific curriculum and training differ between studies, this book is based on practices that are generally regarded as core mindfulness practices among researchers.

Great Idea, But I Don't Have Time

I know what you're thinking. You barely have time to study for the tests themselves. There's a lot to learn in order to take the SAT, ACT, AP Exams, GRE, LSAT, MCAT, or any other test you're taking. Your needs are twofold: to learn content and to master strategy. In addition to the big standardized tests, you probably have lots of upcoming tests in your classes, too.

"You'll be able to study in a shorter period of time, and you'll have more free time as a result."

You may feel overwhelmed just attempting to study materials for these tests. How on earth can you possibly find time to learn general ideas about test-taking itself?

Here's a secret: you can practice mindfulness *while* studying. And doing so will make you more focused and efficient. You'll be able to study in a shorter period of time, and you'll have more free time as a result.

Will I Lose My Edge?

You may fear that you'll lose your motivation and competitive edge using mindfulness. There's a common misconception that meditation is associated with relaxation in contrast to action. You may picture someone sitting cross-legged on a beach blanket in front of the ocean meditating. You might see it as a passive activity — something to do as procrastination instead of studying.

But research shows that mindfulness actually increases competency and enhances performance. In fact, studies have shown that workers who practice mindfulness have measurable increases in productivity.[2] Mindfulness not only doesn't decrease your motivation for success, but it allows you to be more centered and aware. It's actually anxiety that leads to more mistakes and less effectiveness.

The mindfulness approach is not a plan B for those who want to give up on excelling. Quite the contrary, mindfulness is increasingly being used as the go-to tool for high performers.

Motivation to Start Now

This is a book about taking action. Mindfulness is a skill that will add value to your life, and you will build your skill, minute by minute.

You don't need to master the theories and philosophies of mindfulness before you start. This book will provide you with a concrete roadmap, full of step-by-step instructions, you can use to incorporate mindfulness into your studying

2   Cristián Coo and Marisa Salanova, "Mindfulness Can Make You Happy-and-Productive: A Mindfulness Controlled Trial and Its Effects on Happiness, Work Engagement and Performance," *Journal of Happiness Studies* 19, no. 6 (May 2017): 1691–1711, https://doi.org/10.1007/s10902-017-9892-8; Jeremiah Slutsky et al., "Mindfulness training improves employee well-being: A randomized controlled trial," *Journal of Occupational Health Psychology*, 24, no. 1 (2019): 139–149, http://dx.doi.org/10.1037/ocp0000132.

and test-taking routine — the same studying you would do anyway — and start improving your test scores.

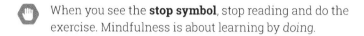

When you see the **stop symbol**, stop reading and do the exercise. Mindfulness is about learning by *doing*.

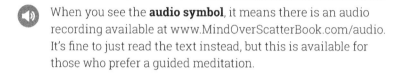

When you see the **audio symbol**, it means there is an audio recording available at www.MindOverScatterBook.com/audio. It's fine to just read the text instead, but this is available for those who prefer a guided meditation.

Now, take your first action: turn the page and dive right in. It's time to boost your test scores, improve your grades, lose the stress, and be happier!

PART I

WHY MINDFULNESS?

CHAPTER 1

WHY YOU MAY NOT BE REACHING YOUR FULL POTENTIAL

L et's explore some problems you may be facing as you gear up for an upcoming test and how a mindfulness approach can help you overcome these problems.

You've Hit a Wall

You've spent hours studying content and learning strategies for an upcoming test. Maybe you've even taken special test prep classes to learn test-taking strategies. You might even have a tutor to help you with all this. But you've hit a wall in your results. The perfect score is still elusive — you're not performing at the level you think you should be, given all the effort you're putting in. Or maybe you are getting that perfect score, but the amount of time it takes you and the negative health consequences aren't worth it.

What you have to know is that your test score is more than the sum of content and strategy. How you take the tests — how focused you are, how you deal with challenges during the test and before the test — all affect that test score.

Ultimately, a test is a mental performance, and it's best to approach it that way. Learning your lines isn't enough. You need to learn *how* to perform, and to do so, it helps to take lessons on high performance.

If there's a gap between where you are at now and your ideal — your ideal scores and your ideal lifestyle — mindfulness can help you create a bridge. Mindfulness is not just a strategy for those suffering from anxiety or stress — it's a way of maximizing anyone's potential.

Thoughts and Emotions About Tests Are Half the Battle

You may find tests stressful for many reasons, including:

- You don't have enough time to study
- Too much depends on the outcome
- You're afraid of failing
- Your family expects you to do well
- You think you are a bad test-taker
- The questions are too hard
- You don't have enough time to finish
- You feel guilty if you don't do well

Many of us have negative associations with tests. Tests are out of our control, and they seem to determine our fate, so that makes them particularly daunting. We're constantly fighting the test itself with thoughts about the test.

Think of all the time and energy you put into merely thinking about tests.

Now, try to list all the emotions you attach to tests — for many students, even the thought of a test can be uncomfortable. An upcoming test can ignite:

- Fear
- Anger
- Shame
- Sadness
- Humiliation
- Anxiety
- Many other emotions

Mindfulness allows you to separate your thoughts and emotions about the test from the test itself. Tests can be challenging enough; you don't need to battle thoughts and emotions about tests on test day, too. Practice mindfulness ahead of time, and you can keep these thoughts and emotions at bay while you focus on the test itself.

Resistance Is Futile

While no one wants to be reduced to a number, tests do just that. Tests allow institutions to make quicker decisions by allowing a score to represent you. It's much more time-consuming and costly to get to know you in a more meaningful and holistic way. So if you feel judged and dehumanized by the testing process, what you're feeling makes sense.

While some high schools and colleges are reducing reliance on tests, the overwhelming testing culture in academic environments — and society at large — is here to stay. Institutions need objective measures of performance. For most high schools and colleges, tests have assumed that role; these institutions rely on grades based on test scores and standardized testing.

In approaching your emotions toward test-taking, it's helpful to acknowledge testing as a fact of life. Accepting it doesn't mean you have to like it or pass moral judgment on it, but it does mean stopping your internal fight against the existence of the tests themselves.

"I hate tests!"

"It's so unfair that I have to take these tests!"

"It's so wrong that my test score will determine what college I go to!"

"Tests are evil!"

Don't waste your energy. Sure, you might be motivated to fight against testing in our culture at some point, but right now, for most of us, tests are a part of life. The present reality is that they matter a lot, and certain opportunities we want are tied to the outcome of these tests.

Sadly, you're not even done with tests after getting into college. In addition to midterms and finals in your college classes, you may also need to take entrance exams to graduate school, law school, medical school and other professional schools; professional licensing tests such as bar exams; employment tests that are part of job interviews, and countless other tests.

You may be operating with the prevailing advice in many high-pressure environments:

"You should just push through and sacrifice your physical and mental health to pass this hurdle." However, following this advice can be damaging, especially when the progression of tests you'll be facing is endless.

Instead of using your thoughts and emotional energy to resist the fact that you have to take tests, or the fact that society will be judging you on the outcome of tests, change the way you study for and take tests instead. Mindfulness can allow you to do that.

Negative Health Consequences

Students today appear more stressed than ever by academic pressure. Why is that? Part of it is the competitiveness of admissions to the most selective schools. As more students apply to more schools, there's a sense of scarcity. There are also limited spots in some of the most desired graduate and professional schools, too.

Also, thanks to social media, we find out more easily what other people are doing. When you hear about all the amazing things other students seem to be doing, all while getting perfect GPAs and perfect standardized test scores, you can get a sinking feeling.

Challenge Success, a research-based organization affiliated with Stanford University, surveyed 43,000 students from high-performing schools and found that three-quarters of high school students and half of middle school students reported "often or always feeling stressed" by their schoolwork.[3] The National Academies of Sciences, Engineering and Medicine added students in "high-achieving schools" to their list of groups "at risk" for elevated levels of chronic stress that can affect health and well-being.[4] The other at-risk groups include kids living in poverty and foster care, recent immigrants, and those with incarcerated parents. While it may seem surprising to put relatively affluent students in the same category as these other vulnerable groups, and the stressors and other life circumstances are certainly different, the effects of chronic stress are still debilitating.

The stress does not let up in college. In a survey of nearly 40,000 college students, the American College Health Association found that 75% of students were suffering from moderate to high levels of stress. In addition, nearly 20% of students reported they were suffering from serious psychological distress.[5]

Stress itself is not inherently bad. It's your physical or emotional response to the demands of life, particularly when they're challenging. A certain amount of stress can actually be healthy — it can gear you up for a challenge — but it

3   Breheny Wallace, "Students In High-Achieving Schools Are Now Named An 'At-Risk' Group, Study Says," *Washington Post*, September 26, 2019, https://www.washingtonpost.com/lifestyle/2019/09/26/students-high-achieving-schools-are-now-named-an-at-risk-group/.

4   National Academies of Sciences, Engineering, and Medicine, "Vibrant And Healthy Kids: Aligning Science, Practice, And Policy To Advance Health Equity" (repr., Washington DC: The National Academies Press, 2019), https://doi.org/10.17226/25466.

5   *American College Health Association-National College Health Assessment III: Undergraduate Student Reference Group Executive Summary* (Silver Spring, MD: American College Health Association, 2020), https://www.acha.org/documents/ncha/NCHA-III_Spring_2020_Undergraduate_Reference_Group_Executive_Summary.pdf.

becomes problematic when it's chronic or you don't balance stress with relaxation and other tools that can help you manage it.

Many students, however, face one stress after another without any time to recover. This chronic stress is not healthy.

You may feel a sense of doom looking at all the things you have to do, everything that is coming up in your schedule. When you don't feel like there is enough time to do everything you need to do and do well, you can get that pressure cooker feeling. Often, students find that they can't possibly get everything done in the day, so they take time out of their evenings, too. Sleep is usually the first to go. There's no time for relaxation or spending free time with family and friends.

And there's no time to balance or recover from the stress.

This dysfunctional behavior has become normalized. Especially in some schools, this behavior may seem not only normal but the only option.

Allowing your body to be subject to intense academic stress without relief is not healthy.

Specific Issues Related to Test-Taking

So here you are, stuck in a high-pressure container of stress and impossible expectations, with not enough time in the day for endless homework assignments, practices, games, and performances. And now: it's time to take a test. Is it any surprise that many students are overcome with a variety of afflictions when it comes to test-taking? As a result, students face many issues:

Test anxiety

Anxiety means worry or fear about what's about to happen. You may feel a general sense of worry, perhaps a nervous flutter in your stomach, every day as you find yourself buried under assignments and upcoming tests. Or maybe you feel a strong sensation of dread that descends upon you as a particular test approaches.

Anxiety expresses itself differently in each person. You may feel it in the form of a headache, stomachache, rapid heartbeat, sweating palms, shallow breathing, or something else. You may not feel anything at all until it hits you the day of the test when you simply freeze or have a panic attack.

Anxiety that expresses itself on test day can be a particularly hard blow. You may find yourself full of nervous jitters, unable to perform at your peak. You may suffer a panic attack during a test, interrupting your progress altogether.

Signs of an anxious test-taker:

- Scoring lower on tests than on homework, quizzes, or practice test scores
- A sense of dread with an approaching test
- Short or irregular breathing, rapid heart rate, sweaty palms
- Fidgeting or restless during tests
- Being easily distracted
- Making careless errors
- Feeling rushed and panicked during tests

This is normal and widespread, and you may not be able to stop it altogether. Thus, your goal is to find a way to manage your anxiety and ease it, if possible. The good news is that mindfulness is particularly helpful for anxiety, as shown in Chapter 3.

If your anxiety is severe or mindfulness does not seem to help you, talk to a trusted adult and consider seeing a professional counselor.

Distracting thoughts

When you're studying, or even while you're taking a test, you may find yourself distracted. In this world of instant notifications and gratification, there's a certain discipline needed to focus on just one task. This is especially hard if that task isn't particularly appealing.

When studying, there are infinite distractions available to you at home or even while studying in a library. Having a phone, laptop, or any Internet connection means you could potentially be doing anything – or everything – at the same time you're supposed to be studying. You can chat with friends, respond to emails, or check out the latest cat videos on YouTube.

By harnessing the power of your attention using mindfulness, you will have the tools you need to overcome distracting thoughts during tests.

Even if you're able to physically chain yourself to your study guide and restrain yourself from Internet access, you still have your own mind. This is the problem with distraction during a test itself. In a test environment, where you have no devices or objects to play with, your own mind can still supply plenty of diversions.

Often, distraction or boredom mask fear – an unwillingness or reluctance to face anxiety, stress, or pain. Your mind doesn't want to deal with all the negative emotions associated with your test, so it directs your attention elsewhere. This is a defense mechanism your mind uses to try to prevent you from being hurt. If you're able to deal with your anxiety, you may find yourself able to settle down and focus more.

Whatever the cause of your distracting thoughts, they will definitely interfere with your test performance. Ideally, you want to direct the maximum amount of attention possible to the test itself. Unrelated thoughts will count against this goal.

By harnessing the power of your attention using mindfulness, you will have the tools you need to overcome distracting thoughts during tests.

Procrastination/avoidance

You may find yourself simply avoiding studying for the test, avoiding thinking about the fact that it's looming because you experience so much negativity associated with it. You may find yourself prioritizing other things over studying for a test and doing absolutely anything — and everything — else.

Procrastinating studying doesn't necessarily mean being unproductive. You could distract yourself from one unpleasant task (upcoming SAT test) by doing homework assignments instead. You may even elect to clean your room.

Mindfulness can help with this, too, as you become aware of your motives and acknowledge what you're doing. Also, once you face the test itself, full-on, you have less to run from. No need to hide. Just acknowledge it is there.

Physical pain

You may suffer from physical symptoms that you don't even associate with the test. As noted above, anxiety frequently manifests as a number of physical symptoms. You may experience pain in your body, an intermittent or constant ache. You may get headaches; others may get stomachaches. An endless number of physical symptoms may actually be stress in disguise.

Of course, you should also always consult your doctor about any medical issues.

Boredom

When you think of exciting things to do, tests are probably not at the top of your list. It's quite possible you might find yourself simply bored. This could happen while studying for a test or even during the test itself. This could be a big problem because it could prevent you from focusing. Often, boredom is a mask for avoidance. Once you use mindfulness to learn how to be engaged by the test itself, you will find boredom less of an issue.

Sleep deprivation

When your life is consumed with studying for a test (along with all your homework, extracurriculars, work, and other commitments), sleep can be the first thing you sacrifice. The American Academy of Sleep Medicine has recommended that teenagers, ages thirteen to eighteen, should sleep eight to ten hours per night, and those older than eighteen should sleep at least seven hours per night on a regular basis. It's not just the number of hours of sleep, though, but the quality of sleep that matters. If you're suffering from anxiety from upcoming stress, it's possible you may have difficulty falling asleep or you wake up in the night with racing thoughts.

Pressure to excel

Even if you don't feel anxiety or stress about the test per se, you may still feel pressure to excel. Most people who read this book are motivated to not only boost their scores but to be better overall.

It's part of our self-improvement-obsessed, high-achieving culture, so it's natural that students, especially those who are in highly competitive environments, would feel this pressure.

You may not recognize this as harmful, and it doesn't have to be. You should just be aware that there is potentially no end to this self-inflicted pressure. It can start with thinking something along the lines of, "I know this is painful and unhealthy, but I just need to get through this one task. Then I'll take care of myself and everything will be okay."

The problem with this approach is that it never ends. The goalposts will always move forward. It doesn't end with college. From standardized tests, college admissions, college grades, and graduate school admission to coveted jobs and so on, there will never be an end to your drive to achieve and excel at the next goal.

Many people discover mindfulness later in life and wish they'd found it sooner. You have an advantage because you're reading this book now. You can use the skills of mindfulness to learn to deal with this pressure whenever you encounter it, whether the pressure comes from family, from schools, or even from yourself.

Clinical Problems

Anxiety and stress from tests are common, and for many students, mindfulness can be an effective way to cope. Mindfulness, however, is not a substitute for medical advice or therapy.

This book does not contain medical advice or diagnosis. You should always consult your doctor for any specific issues relating to your physical or mental health.

COVID-19 Issues

As if academic pressure to excel on tests is not stressful enough under normal circumstances, many of us are still dealing with the effects of a global pandemic. While the ramifications of the pandemic may vary based on where you live and when you're studying, the lingering effect of such a disruption will likely be felt by a lot of people for a long time.

Some institutions may be accepting admissions without test scores, which is a breath of relief. But for most of you, some tests will still be necessary or preferable to make you stand out from the crowd.

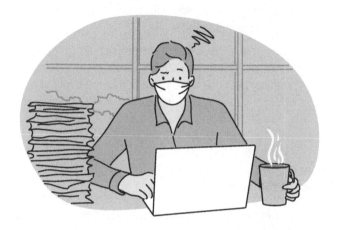

In addition to the negative health effects on those who are directly affected by COVID-19, there has been a sort of pervasive anxiety for all of society. Especially for students, there has been a lot of uncertainty. Missed school and missed events have contributed to a sense of loss, on top of a general feeling of anxiety in the air.

All this can add up to make it harder to focus on academics and tests. A structured study time with a mindfulness focus can be especially helpful during this time. Many of the strategies in this book aimed toward combating anxiety can be helpful for those dealing with COVID-19 issues.

Consider what challenges you're facing while trying to study for and take tests. Can you relate to any of the challenges in this chapter? Is there anything else you're confronting?

Keep these issues in mind as you go through the mindfulness tools later in this book.

What You've Learned

You've identified some of the challenges around tests and test-taking you may be facing, which may include:

✔ Not reaching your full potential because you've hit a wall

✔ Negative thoughts and emotions about tests

✔ Resistance to testing

✔ Stress and other health issues

✔ Test anxiety

✔ Distracting thoughts

✔ Procrastination or avoidance tactics

✔ Physical pain

✔ Boredom

✔ Sleep deprivation

✔ Pressure to excel

✔ Clinical problems

✔ COVID-19 issues

CHAPTER 2

HOW MINDFULNESS CAN HELP

Preparing for a test is so much more than just mastering content and strategy. You also need to prepare your mind, and that's where mindfulness comes in. In this chapter, we'll dive into what exactly mindfulness is, how it works, and why researchers believe mindfulness can help students increase test scores.

What Is Mindfulness?

To be mindful is to be in the present moment. Yes, there's a little more to it than that, but that's the basic concept. You may not have time right now to learn everything about mindfulness. Luckily, that's not necessary for the purpose of using mindfulness for test-taking.

Let's start with a quick exercise.

Take a deep breath.

Ask yourself: What am I thinking about right now?

You may have one or possibly several thoughts running through your mind, even as you're reading this book. If you're like most people, your mind may be in the past or the future.

If it's in the past, you may be thinking of a test you took this morning at school or worrying about something a friend told you at lunch. You may be reminiscing about last summer or thinking about a movie you watched last night.

Or your mind may be in the future instead. Maybe you're feeling hungry and asking yourself what's for dinner? You may be feeling anxious about an upcoming performance or game.

Most of the time, most of us are not fully present. While some of these thoughts are important, they don't serve us well when we're trying to accomplish a task in the present.

For example, if you're reading a reading comprehension passage on a test, wouldn't you want the full benefit of 100 percent of your attention on what you're doing? Do you really want a large percentage of your brain preoccupied with other matters while you're trying to do your best work? Probably not. To avoid that situation during a test, you can use mindfulness as a way to train your brain to be fully present.

When you're fully present while taking a test, you can be aware of any anxious or distracting thoughts that pop into your mind. By becoming aware of these thoughts as they arise, you can avoid letting them derail you or allowing the emotions associated with the thoughts overwhelm you.

Trying to stay in the present moment is one component of mindfulness; the other is that you need to be present in a particular way.

How to Pay Attention

When you practice mindfulness, you learn to pay attention to the present moment in a specific way: with openness and curiosity and without judgment.

Because let's face it: the times we usually do pay attention to the present are when our minds are full of commentary and judgment. This prevents us from focusing on what's actually in front of us.

Let's take the example of Sophia, one of my students who, for a long time, froze whenever it was time to do a math test. She saw the math questions, and her mind was not in the past or the future; her mind was only on that math test just placed on her desk.

Sophia's thoughts: "This is painful. I can't do this. I hate math. This is painful. Math is awful. I hate this. I don't want to be here. I'm going to fail."

> Your goal is to have a single-minded focus on the questions and answer them correctly.

Sophia's mind may have been in the present, but it was also judging the math and making assumptions and commentary triggered by her past experience instead of fully appreciating (and being able to effectively respond to) the questions on the present test. Most of us have this running commentary in our head as we go through life. There's nothing wrong with you if you have these thoughts; mindfulness just trains us to be aware of them so they loosen our grip on us and eventually fade to the background.

Think how much clearer your mind will be on test day when it is not cluttered with thoughts — possibly negative thoughts — about the test as you're taking it. Your goal is to have a single-minded focus on the questions and answer them correctly; thus, you want to discard anything unrelated or distracting. Mindfulness practice will train you on how to do that.

We'll talk more about specific techniques in Part II, but for now, it's important to realize that there are tools you can learn to help control your thoughts.

Mindfulness Versus Meditation

> "There's no need to become an expert at meditation because anyone can use meditation as a tool to become more mindful."

While mindfulness and meditation are often used interchangeably, it's helpful to understand the difference. While meditation can help you practice and cultivate a mindful mind — and for some people is the most effective way to learn mindfulness — you don't need to meditate to practice mindfulness. Mindfulness is just a specific way of paying attention that can be integrated into your daily life while speaking, writing, eating, playing sports, and taking tests. Really, it can be used at any time and in any situation.

If you're reading this book to improve your test performance, your goal should be to become a mindful test-taker.

Meditation is a formal practice, usually sitting, and you don't have all the external stimuli and distractions that you would have while doing your everyday tasks. You're in a quiet space where there's not much distraction, so you can "flex" your mindfulness muscles. It's like doing a workout to train your brain.

The good news is there's no need to become an expert at meditation because anyone can use meditation as a tool to become more mindful.

There are hundreds of types of meditation, but for the purposes of this book, we're focusing on what is known as mindfulness meditation — the type of meditation that facilitates present-moment awareness.

How Mindfulness Works to Bring You into the Present

We've discussed why most of us spend most of our time outside the present and why it is important to be present. But how does mindfulness bring us into the present?

Even while your thoughts are lost in the past or future, a part of you is always in the present moment. Guess what part?

Your body! Your body has nowhere else to go, nowhere else to be, than in the present.

For this reason, many mindfulness practices use the body as an anchor. When you focus your attention on your body, it is one way of getting yourself back to the present moment.

You can use body awareness and breath awareness practices to help you achieve this. For some people, perhaps due to health issues or trauma, it may be difficult being in your body. So there are alternative places you can use as your anchor, as we will discuss in Chapter 5.

Is Mindfulness Religious or Scientific?

Mindfulness meditation is derived from Buddhist practices originating over two thousand years ago. These teachings were brought to the western world in the 1960s, but in the last decade, the popularity of mindfulness has exploded. As mindfulness has become more mainstream, it has transcended its religious roots and become increasingly science-based. Mindfulness meditation, as it is usually practiced in the West, and as it is taught in this book, is secular and does not require any religious belief.

Scientists and researchers are increasingly studying mindfulness in controlled studies and publishing their research in prestigious, peer-reviewed scientific studies. In the next section, we'll go over some of the key findings of the science. The point of understanding the scientific basis of mindfulness is to give you confidence and motivation to learn and use this practice. When you take a look at the science, you can feel confident that mindfulness is not a fad or based on quack science or wishful thinking.

 Reflect on this question: How do you think it would benefit your life if your mind was in the present more often?

What You've Learned

You've identified some of the challenges around tests and test-taking you may be facing, which may include:

✔ Mindfulness means paying attention to the present moment with openness and curiosity and without judgment.

✔ You can practice mindfulness at any time during the day — you don't have to be sitting in meditation.

✔ A good way to access the present moment is by paying attention to your body.

CHAPTER 3

THE SCIENCE BEHIND THE CLAIMS: HOW MINDFULNESS INCREASES TEST SCORES, DECREASES STRESS, AND BOOSTS HAPPINESS

A growing body of research demonstrates the numerous benefits of mindfulness, including test-taking benefits: higher test scores, better focus, improved memory, decreased anxiety, less stress, and more happiness. However, it's important to keep in perspective that mindfulness is a relatively new field. Compared to other areas of research, such as the correlation between exercise and heart disease, mindfulness research is still young. The results are promising, however, and the body of research correlating mindfulness with improved attention and decreased stress is particularly strong.

Science, Don't Care?

Understanding the science supporting mindfulness can inspire and motivate you to try it and stick with the practice. My students are always excited to try mindfulness after they hear about all the positive research. Learning a little about the science, and particularly learning details of specific, relatable studies, can help you create your own internal buy-in for mindfulness.

For me, knowing that mindfulness improves the quality of my sleep helps motivate me to meditate for a few minutes before bed. Even though I'd rather just go to bed, my rational mind tells me I will sleep sooner and better if I just meditate first. When you learn about how mindfulness can impact your test performance and your stress levels, you just may hesitate a little more before skipping a practice.

The research is compelling and motivating, but it's also not essential to know. If you have an upcoming deadline and are short on time, you can skip this chapter and come back to it if you need motivation later on.

Mindfulness and Test Scores

Mindfulness is increasingly being taught and incorporated into schools, validated both by the experience of teachers and the research that shows mindfulness is useful for students.

While most scientific research has focused on the social-emotional benefits of mindfulness, a growing amount of research examines the effect of mindfulness on academic performance.

Researchers have studied the effect of mindfulness practices on test performance and found mindfulness may help boost standardized test scores. In one randomized, controlled trial — the gold standard for clinical studies — students who participated in a two-week mindfulness class had an average improvement of sixteen percentile points on the reading comprehension section of the GRE.[6]

The class met four times each week and required participants to engage in ten to twenty minutes of mindfulness exercises

6   Michael D. Mrazek, et al., "Mindfulness Training Improves Working Memory Capacity and GRE Performance While Reducing Mind Wandering," *Psychological Science* 24, no. 5 (2013): 776–81.

during each class. In addition, students were asked to practice ten minutes of daily meditation outside of class. The mindfulness exercises required focused attention on anchors such as breath and sound (similar to the practices discussed in Chapter 5).

Mindfulness decreases mind-wandering and working memory capacity

How does practicing mindfulness improve test performance? According to the researchers, mindfulness was effective because it helped participants decrease their mind-wandering and increase their working memory capacity. Both of these factors contributed to higher test scores in the participants who practiced mindfulness.

Mind-wandering is a shift of attention from a task to unrelated concerns. It's probably not surprising that mindfulness — which is a practice designed to train one's attention — helps decrease mind-wandering. When the mind wanders less, students can focus better on the test itself. Researchers have also shown that mind-wandering can impair test performance. In a separate study, mind-wandering has been associated with impaired performance on the SAT.[7]

Many other research studies support the correlation between mindfulness practice and improved focus and attention.[8] Given these studies and the nature of mind-wandering, the test score increases are easier to understand. One meta-study reviewed over 4,000 studies of mindfulness and concluded that mindfulness can help keep attention stable and help

7   Michael D. Mrazek et al., "The Role of Mind-Wandering in Measurements of General Aptitude," *Journal of Experimental Psychology: General* 141, no. 4 (2012): 788–98, https://doi.org/10.1037/a0027968.
8   C.G. Jensen et al., "Mindfulness Training Affects Attention—or Is it Attentional Effort?," *Journal of Experimental Psychology: General* 14, no. 1 (2012): 106; Antoine Lutz et al., "Attention Regulation and Monitoring in Meditation," *Trends in Cognitive Sciences* 12, no. 4 (2008): 163–69; Yi-Yuan Tang et al., "Short-Term Meditation Training Improves Attention and Self-Regulation," *Proceedings of the National Academy of Sciences* 104, no. 43 (2007): 17152–56.

one remain focused on the present. Those who completed mindfulness training were better able to remain vigilant and focused, especially on visual and listening tasks.[9]

The role of an improved working memory capacity in improving test scores should also be noted. Working memory is a type of short-term memory that is essential for test-taking. Imagine doing a word problem where you need to keep track of all the background details while you perform calculations. The strength of your working memory allows you to keep all the applicable information in your mind and simultaneously make use of that information and do the necessary math to come up with an answer.

The connection between mindfulness and working memory has also been studied in clinical research. Scientists have found that mindfulness meditators show enhanced working memory performance.[10]

Mindfulness reduces test anxiety

Another way mindfulness helps students score higher on tests is by reducing test anxiety. In one study, researchers asked students to take a math test in a high-pressure environment and found that students with greater mindfulness performed measurably better on the math test. In a second part of the study, researchers also followed students taking a calculus course and found that mindfulness benefited students' performance on high-stakes exams and quizzes during the class. The authors attributed the results to the reduction in test anxiety from mindfulness.[11]

The researchers found that mindfulness allowed students to devote more attention to the test instead of their anxieties,

9   D. J. Good, et al., "Contemplating Mindfulness at Work: An Integrative Review," *Journal of Management* 42, no. 1 (2015): 114, https://doi.org/10.1177/0149206315617003.

10   A. P. Jha et al., "Examining The Protective Effects of Mindfulness Training on Working Memory Capacity and Affective Experience," *Emotion*, 10, no. 1 (2010): 54.

11   D.B. Bellinger, M.S. DeCaro, and P.A. Ralston, "Mindfulness, Anxiety, and High–Stakes Mathematics Performance in the Laboratory and Classroom," *Consciousness and Cognition* 37 (2015):123–32.

which in the absence of mindfulness would have consumed valuable working memory resources. The study authors stated, "Mindfulness may allow students to remain focused on the task in anxiety-producing testing situations. Thus, students with greater mindfulness may be better able to thrive in important testing situations that might otherwise lead to underperformance."[12] The study found that mindfulness training may be an especially useful method for reducing the impact of test anxiety and pressure felt in high-stakes testing situations.

The effect of mindfulness could be seen when students were solving test problems that place a high demand on working memory. Without mindfulness, the feeling of pressure and anxiety disrupted the working memory needed to solve high-demand problems.

This study provides support for the benefit of mindfulness in academic testing situations. However, unlike the GRE research study, where a specific mindfulness class was given to all study participants, this study is based on self-reported measures of mindfulness and anxiety, so it does not provide guidance on specific interventions to support mindfulness.

Mindfulness and Academic Achievement

Researchers have also studied the impact of greater mindfulness on grade point average and standardized test scores. In a study of two thousand middle school students, researchers found that greater mindfulness had a significant correlation with academic achievement, including higher grade point average and higher scores on standardized tests in mathematics and literacy.[13] These results were consistent across demographic characteristics. Researchers

12   D.B. Bellinger, "Mindfulness," 131.

13   Camila Caballero et al., "Greater Mindfulness Is Associated with Better Academic Achievement In Middle School," Mind, Brain, And Education 13, no. 3 (2019): 157–66, doi:10.1111/mbe.12200.

have also found that mindfulness is associated with improved academic performance for students in college and professional schools.[14] While the number of specific studies studying the effect of mindfulness on test scores and academic performance is limited, as most research has focused on social-emotional benefits of mindfulness, a large number of studies show that mindfulness improves the qualities known to be associated with higher test scores: improved attention and focus, improved working memory capacity, and decreased anxiety.

Mindfulness and Stress

The research linking mindfulness practice to the reduction of stress is well established, and the correlation between mindfulness and the body's stress response is very strong. Many scientists believe that there is more than just a correlation — that mindfulness actually decreases stress.[15]

In numerous studies, researchers looked at one or more of the following types of data to find the link between mindfulness and stress:

- Scans of brains (MRI) before and after completion of a mindfulness class
- Scans of brains taken while someone meditates
- Cortisol levels (a hormone associated with stress response) before and after completion of a mindfulness class

14 Gina Paul, Barb Elam and Steven J. Verhulst, "A Longitudinal Study Of Students' Perceptions Of Using Deep Breathing Meditation To Reduce Testing Stresses," Teaching And Learning In Medicine 19, no. 3 (2007): 287–92, doi:10.1080/10401330701366754; Pamela D. Hall, "The Effect Of Meditation On The Academic Performance Of African American College Students," Journal Of Black Studies 29, no. 3 (1999): 408–15, https://doi.org/10.1177/002193479902900305; Olga Vorontsova-Wenger et al., "Relationship Between Mindfulness, Psychopathological Symptoms, And Academic Performance In University Students," Psychological Reports (2020), https://doi.org/10.1177/0033294119899906.

15 Madhav Goyal et al., "Meditation Programs For Psychological Stress And Well-Being," JAMA Internal Medicine 174, no. 3 (2014): 357–68 , doi:10.1001/jamainternmed.2013.13018.

The part of your brain responsible for your stress response is your amygdala. This is also known as the "fight-or-flight" part of your brain, the primitive part your early ancestors relied on to respond to an attack by a saber-toothed tiger. It's your body's natural reaction to perceived danger. Your body releases a series of hormones and adrenaline that prepare your body to either fight the danger or run away from it. Physical signs of the fight-or-flight response can include rapid heartbeat and breathing, pale or flushed skin, and trembling.

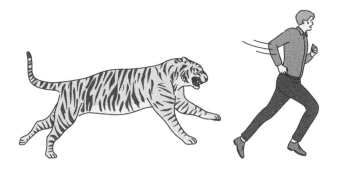

 You probably don't have any saber-toothed tigers lurking around your neighborhood, but you've likely experienced your body reacting as if you were facing one. Think of a time when your body reacted to a situation with fight-or-flight. What physical reactions did you have?

If you find your body in a major state of panic when taking a test, your body is probably just responding the way your ancestors would to that tiger: your heart rate rises, your breathing quickens, your palms sweat, and you start shaking. While those physical reactions may have been appropriate to evade fierce creatures, modern-day stresses usually don't warrant the same response.

Luckily, it's possible to actually change our brains — a concept scientists call neuroplasticity — so we don't trigger the fight-or-flight response every time we encounter a challenging situation. Scientists have found you can actually change — "rewire" — your brain, and mindfulness has been shown to be an effective way to do so.

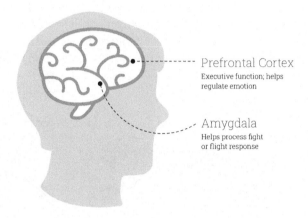

Prefrontal Cortex
Executive function; helps regulate emotion

Amygdala
Helps process fight or flight response

It's beyond the scope of this book to summarize all of the studies on mindfulness and stress. But it is useful to know that scientists have found a substantial correlation between mindfulness and the following:

- A dampening of activity of the amygdala (the fight-or-flight part of the brain).
- An increase in the connections between the amygdala and prefrontal cortex, which is responsible for your executive function, that can help regulate emotion. These connections help you to be less reactive to stressors and to recover better from stress when you experience it.
- A decrease in cortisol levels. When you get stressed, the hormone, cortisol, increases in your body. In research studies of mindfulness, participants engaging in a mindfulness program have been found to have a marked decrease in cortisol levels.

How Long Do You Need to Practice Mindfulness to Get the Benefits?

A recent scientific study conducted at New York University showed that participants had measurable benefits — improved mood, reduced anxiety, and strengthened attention and memory — after eight weeks of practicing for thirteen minutes a day.[16]

The study included forty-two participants who were randomly assigned to either a meditation group or a control group. None of the participants had a previous meditation practice. Each day, the meditation group listened to a thirteen-minute recording of a guided meditation that included breathing exercises and full-body scans (similar to the practices in Chapter 5). The meditation also included a time of silence where subjects could meditate on their own. The control group was given a daily podcast of the same length to listen to. The podcast included cultural and current interest topics, but did not discuss any meditation practices.

Each week, the participants took mood questionnaires and were tested on cognitive tasks. Their cortisol levels were also measured. The study showed that eight weeks of daily brief meditation measurably improved mood, reduced anxiety in response to stress, and improved aspects of attention and memory. The control group did not show these same results. Thus, the authors concluded that meditative effects are cumulative and only emerge with repeated practice over time.

There are limitations to this study, including the relatively small number of participants. And, it's important to know that other studies (such as the study showing increases in GRE scores) required only two weeks to show results in test-

16 Julia C. Basso et. al., "Brief, daily meditation enhances attention, memory, mood, and emotional regulation in non-experienced meditators," *Behavioural Brain Research* 236, no. 1 (January 2019): 208–20.

taking. So it is certainly possible that even if you have less than eight weeks, you can see results.

That said, this study does provide helpful guidance to help you determine an optimal amount of time to practice. Thirteen minutes a day is doable. Most research studies show that the beneficial effects are cumulative — the more consistently you practice, the more benefits you get. Interestingly, it is likely more important to practice daily than to increase the length of your sessions.

Mindfulness Can Change Your Brain in Eight Weeks

Other research has shown that the brain undergoes measurable changes — some areas shrink and others expand — as a result of mindfulness meditation. A landmark study conducted in 2011, which has been followed by additional studies confirming the results, showed that mindfulness meditation can create these brain changes in as little as eight weeks. In this study, researchers took MRI scans (brain scans) of new meditators prior to and after a mindfulness training program, where participants practiced meditation for an average of twenty-seven minutes a day.[17]

In this book, you'll learn how to combine your mindfulness time with study time. This will make eight weeks of practice — or more — within reach for most students.

How Mindfulness Can Make You Happier

Scientists have found that one of the leading causes of unhappiness is mind-wandering — not paying attention to what you are doing.

---

17 Britta K Hölzel et al., "Mindfulness Practice Leads to Increases in Regional Brain Gray Matter Density," *Psychiatry Research: Neuroimaging* 191, no. 1 (2011): 36–43. https://doi.org/10.1016/j.pscychresns.2010.08.006.

Imagine being miserable in Disneyland — the happiest place on earth. You know you have an upcoming test on Monday, a super important test that you're convinced will determine your GPA. You had already planned this trip, so you go to Disneyland anyway. But every minute you wait in line is agonizing. You can't stop feeling stressed out and worried about the upcoming test. Every bite of Dole Whip and crunch of churros is accompanied by guilt. How dare you enjoy these treats when you should be studying? Seeing all the laughing, happy people around you makes you feel worse.

While being miserable in Disneyland might seem to be a rare occurrence, it's actually common for people to be unhappy while engaging in a pleasant activity. Scientists have found that your likeliness of happiness is not tied to what type of activity you are engaging in, but rather how present you are while engaging in the activity.

A study by Harvard researchers Matthew Killingsworth and Daniel Gilbert found that only 4.6% of a person's happiness is attributable to the specific activity they are doing at the time. The study tracked 2,250 subjects, checking in with them at random times (via a mobile app) and asking them to record what they were doing at the moment and what their mind was focused on. The researchers concluded that people's attention was not on the task they were doing more than 47% of the time and that this mind-wandering was the cause of their unhappiness, not the consequence.[18]

As Killingsworth stated, "Mind-wandering is an excellent predictor of people's happiness. In fact, how often our minds leave the present is a better predictor of our happiness than the activities in which we're engaged."[19] This study shows that when we're lost in thoughts and worries about the past or anxiety about the future, we're not able to truly experience a pleasant experience — not even Disneyland.

18 Matthew A Killingsworth and Daniel T. Gilbert. "A Wandering Mind Is an Unhappy Mind," *Science* 330, no. 6006 (2010): 932.
19 Steve Bradt, "Wandering Mind Not A Happy Mind," *The Harvard Gazette*, November 11, 2010, https://news.harvard.edu/gazette/story/2010/11/wandering-mind-not-a-happy-mind/.

The opposite is also true. You can be happy even while engaging in activities you dislike or regard as unpleasant, such as washing the dishes or cleaning a bathroom. If you take the effort to immerse yourself fully in whatever you're doing — feeling the soap bubbles on your hands as you're cleaning the dishes or observing the contours of the bathroom tiles as you wipe them clean — you'll find that you can be happy even in the midst of these activities.

So science has proven that we are not doomed to misery — or destined for happiness — based merely on our circumstances. We each have the power in our minds, the power of our attention, to find happiness in each moment, no matter how boring or painful the activity we're engaged in. It's not as easy as it sounds, though. There's no magic potion or spell to create this transformation. Being present is a skill that needs to be learned and diligently practiced.

Positive Emotions

In addition to the happiness that comes from focusing on a task, mindfulness practices can help you directly cultivate positive emotions. Practices such as self-compassion and gratitude, which you will learn in Chapter 8, work by giving your brain practice in experiencing these emotions. By repeatedly having the experience of positive emotions, your brain rewires to experience these more frequently, even when you are not doing these practices.

Scientific studies have shown that cultivating gratitude can have many psychological benefits, including improving mental performance.[20] Higher levels of gratitude have also been associated with changes in the brain, such as greater neural sensitivity in the medial prefrontal cortex, a brain area associated with learning and decision-making.

20   Robert A. Emmons and Michael E. McCullough, The Psychology of Gratitude (New York: Oxford University Press, 2004).

What You've Learned

✔ Studies link mindfulness with improved test scores, grades, and academic performance.

✔ Studies link mindfulness with a reduction in stress and other health benefits.

✔ Scientists have shown that your brain can measurably change after practicing mindfulness.

✔ Mindfulness can make you happier because it helps you focus on the present.

✔ Mindfulness can rewire your brain so you feel positive emotions more often.

PART II

SIX MINDFUL STEPS

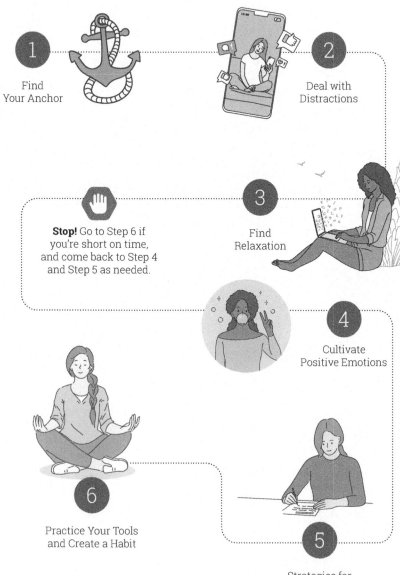

STEPS TO LEARN
MINDFULNESS

1 Find Your Anchor

2 Deal with Distractions

Stop! Go to Step 6 if you're short on time, and come back to Step 4 and Step 5 as needed.

3 Find Relaxation

4 Cultivate Positive Emotions

6 Practice Your Tools and Create a Habit

5 Strategies for Stress and Difficult Emotions

CHAPTER 4

YOUR ROAD MAP

After learning about the scientific research on the benefits of mindfulness, you're probably eager to try it out for yourself.

Since you have hundreds of possible mindfulness practices to choose from, the choice can be overwhelming. Do you really need more decisions? How will you know which mindfulness practices are grounded in science and which are just promoted for clickbait? How will you know which ones to try first?

The good news is that I've done the heavy lifting for you. Based on the scientific research on mindfulness, Part II will provide you a step-by-step guide on what practices to learn, while providing options along the way if something doesn't seem to be working well for you.

Preparing Yourself: Space, Posture and Expectations

First, let's start with the basics of setting up your space and your expectations.

Before you start trying out mindfulness practices, read this section so you can prepare the stage for success and avoid common misconceptions and pitfalls.

You don't have to sit on a remote mountaintop to meditate. Nope. Find a spot that's comfortable and easily accessible to you.

You can sit on a chair or on the floor, but be sure your back can be upright and not too relaxed. Feel free to use pillows or cushions to prop up your legs so you can be comfortable.

A sofa or bed may make you too relaxed and sleepy. So, especially as you first start out, lying down or reclining while meditating may not be the best option. For mindfulness meditation, you want to be alert, not sleepy.

If possible, find somewhere that is quiet and doesn't have too many distractions.

Put down this book, and find a place. It may not be perfect — it may not even be quiet or comfy — but finding any place is better than not starting.

It's useful to meditate in the same place every day. You'll start to associate that spot with meditation, and your body may even initiate the process of getting you primed for meditation as soon as you head toward that spot.

Remember, this book is not about creating a meditation practice just for the fun of it — you want to develop mindfulness to help you boost your test scores. So, in addition to finding a quiet space to hone your mindfulness skills, you should also, as soon as possible, start practicing "in the room where it happens." You may not be able to go to the testing center in advance, but you can try practicing in your classroom or library or desk where you study at home. If it's in a public place, it's fine to keep your eyes open if you don't feel comfortable closing your eyes.

This studying/testing place doesn't have to be the place you practice every day (in fact, it's best to find a quiet, comfortable place for that), but it's good to occasionally practice in those places too, so you can start to associate mindfulness with the place where you're studying/taking your test.

What to Know Before You Start

Your mind will wander—and that's okay

When you sit down and focus on any one thing — whether it's your breath in meditation or a math problem while studying — it's natural that your mind will wander to other thoughts or topics. That's what our minds do. It's normal. Mindfulness practice just asks that you be aware each time your mind does this. You don't have to direct your mind to stop wandering or get frustrated each time it does. Simply acknowledge that your mind has wandered, and gently bring your attention back to the object of your focus.

It is the act of being aware that your mind has wandered and bringing it back, over and over again, that builds your mindfulness muscle. So, when you find that you've been lost in distraction, realize that you are succeeding — not failing — at mindfulness. The important thing is that you have an awareness of what is going on in your mind.

An empty mind is not the goal

One of the biggest misconceptions about mindfulness is that the goal is to empty your mind of all thoughts, and then you will somehow achieve a state of bliss when this happens. Unfortunately, this myth keeps a lot of people from meditating at all.

"Meditation is not for me," my friend's daughter told me when I invited her to join a mindfulness class. "I have way too many thoughts. There's no way I can clear my mind."

Mindfulness is like a laser beam that brings attention to what is in your mind. The more thoughts you have, the more opportunities you have to practice and learn mindfulness. It allows you to be aware of the very fact that you are distracted. Science shows that this awareness itself, practiced over time, will gradually allow you to focus more on the tasks in front of you.

Bring your curiosity

You may be thinking that sitting down with your eyes closed sounds boring. Here's a secret: if you bring an attitude of curiosity toward your object of attention, it can actually be fascinating. For example, take your breath. You've literally been breathing every moment of your life, since birth. But it's not often, if ever, that we take the time to really examine our breathing. Do we breathe fast or slow? Are our breaths deep or shallow? What happens to the rest of our body as we breathe? Does it cause movement elsewhere? Bringing curiosity to the process can transform this practice into something you enjoy.

If you still can't convince yourself to do this, refresh yourself on Chapter 3. Paying attention to your breathing has been scientifically proven to have innumerable benefits, however dull it may seem.

Be kind to yourself

We've established that you want to do well in school and other areas of your life. While it's great to be a high achiever, sometimes you may be hard on yourself when you don't meet your goals. In fact, it's common for goal-oriented students first learning meditation to be so focused on "succeeding" and getting it right that they judge themselves harshly when they think they've failed.

The good news is that you can't fail at meditation. Really. Remember, the more thoughts and distractions you have during your meditation, the more opportunities you actually have to practice.

Meditation shouldn't be one more thing you have to judge yourself about, so be kind to yourself. It sounds kind of cheesy, I know, but you've taken a huge step just by reading this book — so direct some kindness toward yourself as you learn this new skill.

There's no correct way to breathe

Ever since you first started school, adults have probably been telling you the "right" way to do things and admonishing you when you fail. When some people come to meditation, they're eager to learn the "right" way to breathe and then ready to work hard to breathe that way.

While some specific breathing techniques exist to help you relax (see Chapter 7), in mindfulness meditation there is no "correct" way to breathe. In fact, if you force yourself to breathe in a certain way, you're missing the point. Mindfulness, at its heart, is being with the present moment as it *actually* is, not how you wish it to be.

So breathe naturally, whatever that is for you at the moment. It will change each time you meditate. And, you'll find directing your attention to your breath may affect your breathing too — often, breathing becomes more regular and steady when we pay attention to it. If that's the case, notice and pay attention to the changes.

It's also possible that bringing attention to your breath can make your breath faster and more irregular. For some people, your breath may even be a source of anxiety. And that's okay, too. Notice what's happening to your breath as you focus on it. If bringing attention to your breath brings you more discomfort or anxiety than you can handle, choose another anchor for your practice. I provide you with options in Chapter 5.

Stick with it

The first time I tried to meditate, nothing happened. I had read books and heard lectures about how amazing meditation was supposed to be. But nothing happened.

Let's face it, we live in a society of instant gratification. If reading about all the scientific benefits of mindfulness convinces you to try this out, you may have an image of yourself trying it out and immediately reaping all the benefits.

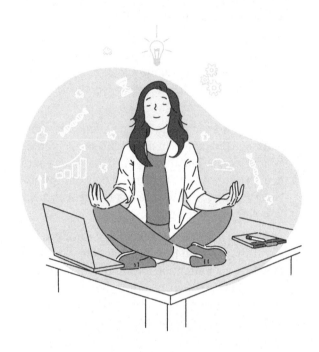

Ah, if only life worked that way. Similar to changes in diet or exercise, benefits come slowly and over time.

While even a few minutes of mindfulness can have a real effect on your body, it's unlikely you'll notice it right away. It can be kind of anticlimactic. You did the research, bought this book, got all set up, and actually meditated! And then nothing happened. No confetti, no drumroll, no sensation of bliss.

When this happens, it's important to remember the research. Remember that the evidence of mindfulness has been scientifically studied and validated. Remember that research shows that the greatest benefits come from *consistent*, *daily* practice.

So try not to be frustrated if you don't experience immediate results. And don't give up.

Simply follow the steps in the upcoming chapters. In each step, you'll acquire tools to add to your Mindfulness Toolbox. Remember, your toolbox doesn't have to be full — you just need to pick the tools you need. Each chapter will explain what those are.

Steps to Learn Mindfulness

Step 1   Find Your Anchor. Gain one or more of these tools: focus practices with breath, body, or sound anchors.

Step 2   Deal with Distractions. Gain one or more of these tools: labeling thoughts, naming emotions, or greet your visitors.

Step 3   Find Relaxation. Gain one or more of these tools: box breathing, waterfall breathing, or belly breathing.

STOP   Go to Step 6 if you're short on time, and come back to Step 4 and Step 5 as needed.

Step 4   Cultivate Positive Emotions. Gain one or more of these tools: smile and breathe, self-compassion, or gratitude.

Step 5   Strategies for Stress and Difficult Emotions. Gain one or more of these tools: STOP, RAIN, or visualization.

Step 6   Practice Your Tools and Create a Habit. The more you practice, the more natural mindfulness will feel to you and the easier it will be to make it part of your routine.

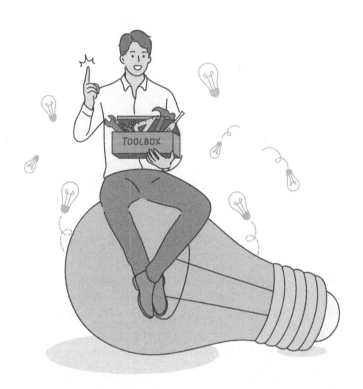

Your Mindfulness Toolbox

As you go through the steps to learn mindfulness, you'll acquire tools to add to your Mindfulness Toolbox.

Once you've learned a tool listed below, check the box next to it. In the last column, write down your favorite option to use. To get a printable version of the toolbox, go to **www. MindOverScatterBook.com/toolbox**

Practices	Tools	Preferences/Notes
Find Your Anchor	☐ Breath ☐ Body ☐ Sounds	
Deal with Distractions	☐ Label Thoughts ☐ Name Emotions ☐ Greet Visitors	
Strategies for Stress and Difficult Emotions	☐ STOP ☐ RAIN ☐ Visualization	
Relaxation Practices	☐ Belly Breathing ☐ Box Breathing ☐ Waterfall Breathing	
Positive Emotions	☐ Smile and Breathe ☐ Self-Compassion ☐ Gratitude	
Practice	☐ Two-Week Plan ☐ Two-Day Plan	

After you go through the steps in the chapters in Part II and fill up your Mindfulness Toolbox, I will give you suggestions on how to practice and master the skills you've just learned. Then, in Part III, you'll learn how to apply these tools to the practice of test-taking.

To practice the tools, read the instructions first and then try them out. Or you can ask a friend or family member to read the instructions to you.

As a reminder, if you prefer a guided meditation, you can find audio recordings for the practices marked with 🔊 at www. MindOverScatterBook.com/audio

What You've Learned

✔ How to prepare your space for mindfulness.

✔ What to expect if you take up mindfulness.

✔ There are six steps you can follow to learn the basics of mindfulness.

✔ By following the steps in the next six chapters, you'll fill in your Mindfulness Toolbox.

CHAPTER 5

STEP ONE — FIND YOUR ANCHOR

> "Focus and simplicity . . . once you get
> there, you can move mountains."
>
> — STEVE JOBS

You have your space set up, and you know what to expect. Now it's time to focus. This chapter will remove all the guesswork for you and make it easy to learn the basic mindfulness tools of focus practices.

Your first step is to find an anchor. An anchor is what you focus on during meditation. It's where you direct your attention and the place where you bring your attention back to after you get distracted.

You have three options for your anchor: your breath, your body, and sounds. These anchors are commonly used in clinical research on mindfulness.

If you're short on time, start with the first option (breath). If that works for you, you can simply choose that, check the breath tool in your Mindfulness Toolbox, and move on to Chapter 6. If it doesn't work, or if you have more time and are curious to experiment, try the other two anchors, too.

I'll refer to the tools in this section as "focus practices."

Anchor Tool 1: Breath

The breath is the most common anchor used for mindfulness meditation. It's always with you, and for most people, it's easy to feel in your body.

Let's start with a simple practice to focus on your breath.

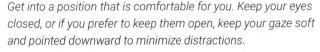

Get into a position that is comfortable for you. Keep your eyes closed, or if you prefer to keep them open, keep your gaze soft and pointed downward to minimize distractions.

Start with a few deep breaths in and out. Fill your lungs fully for each inhale and then exhale everything out. Inhale deeply. Now, exhale everything out.

Now, let your breath settle back into its natural breathing pattern. In mindfulness practices, you don't need to change your breath in any way. There's no right or wrong way to breathe; there's no special way to breathe. You just want to let your breath be the way it is naturally, and keep your attention focused on your breath.

Start by noticing your breath in your nostrils. Bring all your attention and curiosity to your breath. You may notice your breath is cool or warm. You may notice your breath is short or long, deep or shallow. As you inhale, know that you're inhaling. As you exhale, know that you're exhaling.

Next, notice your breathing in your chest. Notice your chest expanding and contracting. Notice if your breath is short or long, deep or shallow. Be aware of any other sensation you feel in your chest, maybe even in your back, as you breathe in and out.

Now, bring your attention to your breath in your stomach. Notice your stomach rising and falling with each breath. Be aware of whether your breath is long or short, deep or shallow.

Ask yourself: Where do you feel your breath the strongest? In your nostrils? In your chest? In your stomach area? If you can't decide, pick one.

Now, bring all your attention to this place in your body where you feel your breath the strongest. Be really curious. What is this breath like? How are you breathing? Try to keep your attention with each inhale and exhale. Continue for a few more breaths (or longer if you're doing a longer practice).

That's it. You've brought attention to your breath and used your breath as an "anchor." If your eyes are closed, you can open them now.

How did it feel to focus on your breath? For the majority of people, the breath works well as an anchor. The breath is always with you and uniquely connects your mind to your body.

However, for some people, breath does not work. For these people, directing attention to their breath can make them feel anxious or even hyperventilate, or it's uncomfortable or difficult for some other reason. If that's the case for you, please move on to Anchor Tool 2 — Body.

You can try the practice again and gradually attempt to expand the amount of time you focus on your breath to one minute and longer.

If focusing on your breath felt neutral or pleasant for you, I recommend you use breath as your primary anchor.

Tool 1 Variation: Counting Breaths

If you're comfortable with using breath as an anchor, you can also try this variation of Tool 1.

This is a great exercise to do if you feel meditation is too open-ended for you. Giving yourself a concrete task to do during the meditation (counting) can help ground you.

While keeping your attention on your breath, make a soft mental note to yourself of the number of breaths you're taking.

Each time you inhale and exhale, count one, like this:

Inhale, exhale — one

Inhale, exhale — two

Inhale, exhale — three

And so on, until you reach ten. If you find yourself distracted away from your breath or lost in a thought, go back to one.

If you can go all the way up to ten without getting distracted (which is not easy), then go back to one. This is not a challenge to see how you far can get. You will always return to one, even after you reach ten.

Remember, don't count aloud and don't let the counting be your primary focus. Your main focus should still be on your breath and the sensations of breathing. The counting should be in the background.

Anchor Tool 2: Body

Now, let's try another anchor: your body. For this anchor, focus your attention on the sensations of your body. For many of us, that's a foreign concept. Some of you, such as dancers and athletes, may be more used to paying attention to your body. Even then, the focus is often on the exterior — positioning and movement. Mindfulness asks you to look deeply inward: what are all the sensations that you can feel within your body?

Experienced meditators develop the ability to experience subtle sensations in their body — some can even feel their internal organs! But that's not necessary to reap the benefits of mindfulness for test-taking.

Can you feel your hands while clapping? Great. We'll start with that and then expand to feel other parts of your body.

The following exercises guide you to experience your body, which is a perfect way to ground yourself in the present moment and away from anxious thoughts.

Option 1: Clapping

In this first activity, you take an active approach to creating a strong sensation in your body — by clapping.

What to do: clap your hands hard, five times.

Then, keep your hands outstretched, palms up, in front of you. You can rest them on a table or your lap.

Focus your attention on your hands. Notice what you feel there. Is there warmth, pain, pressure, tingling, or anything else?

If you don't feel anything, that's okay. Just keep your attention on your hands.

What do you feel now? Is the temperature or pressure changing? Are your hands cooling down, or is the sensation of pain easing?

See if you can keep your attention on your hands for one minute. If you find your attention wanders — as it probably will — just note that it has wandered and gently bring it back to your hands.

By creating a blunt sensation from clapping, you can notice your body more easily than if you're staying still, so this is a good activity to start with. After you have experience with noticing characteristics in your body from the clapping activity (warmth, pressure, etc.), you can move to using your feet as an anchor.

Option 2: Feet

In this activity, you can practice noticing more subtle sensations.

Sit comfortably on a chair with your feet on the floor. Close your eyes, if that feels comfortable for you.

Bring all your attention to your feet. How do you know your feet are there without looking?

Start by feeling your feet on the floor. Can you feel the hardness of the ground underneath you? Can you feel the texture of your socks or your shoes against your skin? Can you feel the pressure of your weight pressing into the ground?

Do you feel any sensations inside your feet? Any tingling, any discomfort, any pressure? Do your feet feel numb? Do you feel coolness or warmth?

It's okay if you don't feel anything. Just try to keep your attention on your feet.

If you can't feel any sensations, try gently wiggling your toes. Does that movement bring any sensations to your feet?

While you do this, other thoughts and sensations may be popping into your head. Maybe you're thinking, "This is so silly. Why am I doing this?" Or maybe: "I'm hungry." Or maybe you're feeling sensations elsewhere, such as noticing a pain in your wrist.

When this happens, just acknowledge the distraction and gently bring your attention back to your feet. In this exercise, your feet are your anchor.

Continue for a minute and then, if your eyes are closed, open them.

Why pay attention to your feet?

For most people, feet are a neutral object of attention. If you have foot pain or an injury, this may not be the case for you. Generally, however, it's a quick way to ground your attention away from distracting or anxious thoughts to the present moment. If for any reason your feet don't work for you as a "neutral" place, pick another place in your body — perhaps your hands. By neutral, you want to locate a part in your body that doesn't elicit a strong physical or emotional response, either positive or negative.

During test-taking, most of you will be sitting on a chair with your feet resting on the ground.

If you find yourself anxious with spiraling thoughts, bringing your attention to your feet is a great way to quickly focus again on the present.

Your feet will always be with you; you don't need to take anything special along with you to have this mindfulness practice handy during a test.

Option 3: Body Scan

Here is a longer practice that is great for practicing mindfulness using body sensations, and it can also be very relaxing.

What are possible sensations you may feel in your body? These examples give you an idea of what to look for:

- Tightness
- Pressure
- Hardness
- Softness
- Tingling
- Throbbing
- Pulsing

- Shivering
- Warmth
- Coolness
- Heaviness
- Lightness
- Anything else you feel

Being familiar with these terms will help you bring awareness to the sensations of your body, but remember, these are just examples. You may feel a sensation that's not on the list — or you may feel nothing at all.

Get yourself in a comfortable position — your back should be upright but not tense, your body relaxed and alert. Close your eyes, if that feels comfortable to you; otherwise, keep them open and your gaze soft and pointed downward.

Take a few deep breaths. Now, let your breath return to its natural rhythm.

Start by noticing your feet. Bring all your attention to your feet. Notice any sensations you feel there.

Now, bring your attention to your legs, notice any sensations you feel in your legs. If you don't feel anything at all, that's okay. Just keep your attention on your legs.

Now, bring your attention to your knees. Slowly move up to your thighs. Feel any sensations that may be in your thighs.

While you're doing this exercise, remember to keep breathing. Breathe naturally. There's no special way you need to breathe. And if thoughts come up — and they will — as soon as you become aware that you've been distracted, gently bring your attention back to your body.

Now, bring your attention to where your body is touching your chair or the ground. This could be in your seat, your thighs, your lower back. Notice where the points of contact are between your body and the chair or the floor. Be aware of any sensations you feel. Do you feel the hardness of the chair beneath you? The warmth of the place where your body touches the chair? Do you feel the softness of your clothes against you?

Keep breathing as you do this.

Now bring your attention up to your stomach. Many people feel tension and hold tightness in their stomach. If you find there is any tightness, or any discomfort there, invite your body to release it. If it's not possible, it's okay. Just be aware of whatever sensations are there.

Bring your attention up from your stomach to your chest. Notice your breath in your chest, and feel the sensation of your chest expanding and contracting. Do you feel any other sensations in your chest area? You don't need to change anything, just notice what's there.

Now, bring your awareness to your back. Your lower back, your middle back, your upper back. We often don't pay much attention to the back of our body. Notice any sensations that are in your back. What do you feel there? If you don't feel anything at all in your back, that's okay too. Just be aware that you're not feeling anything.

Remember to keep breathing.

Now it's time to bring your awareness to your shoulders. What do you feel in your shoulders? This is another place where many people feel tightness or tension. If you feel this, invite your body to soften and release that tension. If that doesn't happen, that's okay. Just be aware of what is there in your shoulders right now.

Bring your attention to your arms. Notice any sensations in your arms. Do you feel heaviness, lightness, tingling, throbbing, or anything else? Now, bring your attention down your arms to your hands and fingers. Do you feel coolness, warmth, pulsing, or any other sensations?

Slowly move your attention to your neck. What do you feel in your neck? Do you feel any sensation there? Keep breathing. Bring your attention to your face. Notice your mouth, your nose, your eyes. Notice your jaw.

Now, bring your attention to your head and your scalp. Do you feel any sensations in this area? If you don't notice anything, just keep your attention at the top of your head for a few moments.

Take a deep breath. If your eyes are closed, slowly open them.

The body scan is a popular mindfulness practice. If you found it helpful, you can repeat this with your own internal guidance. The words above are just suggestions.

You can feel free to try this practice on your own, scanning your body from bottom to top, or top to bottom, making a mental note of the different areas of your body. Some people prefer body scans that go through your body more generally (from the head and neck, to shoulders and torso, to legs and feet), while others prefer to name each specific body part. The more detailed you are, the easier it is to get distracted, so my recommendation is to start with a relatively quicker body scan.

As you get more practice, you can spend more time bringing your awareness to each specific body part (your thumbs, your toes), and even notice more subtle sensations, such as those in your internal organs.

Anchor Tool 3: Sounds

Using outside sounds as your anchor is the third option. This is great for everyone to try, but it's especially helpful if it doesn't feel comfortable to focus inside your body. This is also a practice where you don't need to be in a quiet place.

For this tool, pay attention to the qualities of the sounds you hear — their volume, pitch, and tone. Also, notice how sounds come and go. You don't need to identify the sources of the sounds.

Close your eyes, if that feels comfortable for you, or keep your eyes pointed downward, so you can focus on your hearing.

Notice any sounds around you. If you don't hear anything, be aware of the silence. Listen closely and notice what you hear.

Do you hear voices? Wind? The hum of an air conditioner or heater? Traffic outside?

When you notice a sound, try not to create a story around it. For this exercise, it doesn't matter where the sound is coming from or what it means.

Just observe the qualities of the sound: is it loud or quiet? Ongoing or intermittent? Is it high-pitched or low-pitched? Be aware of when it stops.

If there are multiple sounds, take time to observe each one as it comes and goes.

When you find yourself distracted from the sounds, thinking of something else, gently bring your attention back to the sounds.

Keep listening and observing for two minutes, or as long as you want the session to last.

That's it. You've now learned mindfulness of sounds. Try doing this in noisy places and experiment with keeping your eyes open and closed. This tool teaches you that noises don't have to be a distraction — they can actually help you focus if viewed in the right way.

Choosing Your Anchor

Now that you've practiced bringing your attention to different objects — your breath, your body, and sounds — it's time to choose which anchor is easiest for you to focus on.

If focusing on your breath didn't cause you any discomfort, stick to your breath. That's the tried-and-true anchor of meditation for most people. If you preferred bringing your attention to your feet or another part of your body or the sounds outside, you can use those instead of breath for your focus practices.

Go to the Mindfulness Toolbox now, and put a check mark next to the tools you've completed. Also, write down your preferred choice of anchor. The Mindfulness Toolbox is located at the end of Chapter 4.

CHAPTER 6

STEP TWO — DEALING WITH DISTRACTIONS

> "Distraction wastes our energy, concentration restores it."
>
> — SHARON SALZBERG

Now that you've chosen what you want to focus on, it's time to explore what your mind will end up doing instead. Most likely, thoughts will pop up. Emotions may arise. Physical sensations will appear. How do you combat these distractions and stay focused?

Your second step in learning mindfulness requires you to try out three tools for dealing with distractions. You'll need Tool 1 and Tool 2 for sure, as thoughts and emotions are likely to come up as you try to focus.

Tool 3 provides an alternative way to deal with distractions. Try this out, too, but only add it to your toolbox if it works for you.

If you're short on time, just stick with Tool 1 and Tool 2.

Tool 1: Labeling Thoughts

When you try to focus on your anchor, it's normal that you will start thinking. You may think about your to-do list, about your friends, about dinner, about anything and everything.

After all, our minds are designed to think. It's normal for it to be hard to focus just on your anchor, especially when you first start.

Let's try this next practice to see what you should do when thoughts arise. The following activity is scripted for breath, but if you're choosing a different anchor, focus on that instead of your breath.

Get yourself into a comfortable position and take a few breaths. Close your eyes, if that is comfortable for you. Bring your attention to your breath. Your full, complete attention. Breathe naturally. Just be with your breath, however it is right now. When you inhale, be aware that you are inhaling. When you exhale, be aware that you are exhaling. Notice the sensations of your breath in the place you feel it strongest — in your nostrils, in your chest or in your stomach.

Now, if you are like most people, before long, you'll find yourself distracted in thoughts. You may be lost in a daydream. You may be thinking of something that happened to you yesterday. You may be planning your to-do list for tomorrow.

As soon as you realize this has happened, make a soft mental note, "Thinking," and go back to your breath. Keep doing this over and over again. Don't get frustrated with yourself, as this is how you learn mindfulness. You build your mindfulness muscle every time you become aware that you've been distracted by thoughts.

Try this for one to two minutes the first time you try this practice.

Tool 2: Name Emotions

When you try to meditate, an emotion may arise and distract you from your anchor. It's good to experience this during meditation because the very same thing can happen when you're trying to study for or actually taking a test.

You may feel anxious, panicked, sad, angry, bored, restless, or any other emotion. Both positive and negative emotions can arise. Whether pleasant or unpleasant, an emotion sure can be distracting. What to do?

Initially, the best response is to acknowledge the emotion, just as you would a distracting thought. Name it. "Anger." "Boredom." Whatever it is, name it and acknowledge it. Then, go back to your anchor.

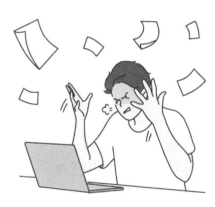

UCLA professor and psychiatrist, Dr. Daniel Siegal, uses the phrase, "name it to tame it," to describe how naming an emotion can help you control your response to the emotion. By naming the emotion, you activate your executive brain (the part of your brain associated with language), which can help calm down the part of your brain responsible for an emotional response.

Take a deep breath.

1. **Ask yourself:** *What am I feeling now?*

2. **Say it aloud.** *Say whatever you're feeling — relaxed, happy, stressed, sad, neutral, angry. Just name it.*

3. **Notice how you feel.** *If you had a strong emotion, notice the effect that naming it had on you (if any).*

4. **Try a focus practice from Chapter 5 (breath, body, or sound).** *If any emotions come up during the practice, try naming them and observe what happens in your body afterward.*

Sometimes, however, an emotion will be so strong and dominant that it simply won't go away. It demands your attention immediately. In this case, when the emotion is hampering your ability to do your task, you need to direct your attention to the emotion itself. If this is the case, try sitting with your emotions as "visitors" in your home, as described in the next practice.

Tool 3: Greet Your Visitors

This tool is useful for dealing with distractions that come in all forms — thoughts, emotions, or a variety of other things. It's also a great practice if you like to use your imagination.

Imagine you live in a house. Thoughts, emotions, and anything else that calls your attention away during studying or tests are merely visitors. They don't live in your house, and you don't have to let them in. It helps, though, to answer the door and acknowledge them; otherwise, they'll keep ringing the doorbell and distract and annoy you.

Your task is to name and acknowledge your visitors. When you become familiar with the identities of your visitors, you can address them easily before they blow up into something unmanageable — such as freezing or having a panic attack during a test.

What type of visitors can you have?

Some visitors can simply be distractions — thinking about what's going to happen in the next episode of a Netflix show. Other visitors can be negative thoughts — doubt or fear, for example. Even positive thoughts can be distracting: excitement about an upcoming party, for example. Visitors can also be physical sensations, such as throbbing pain or a tight back, which grab your attention away from your anchor.

When you practice mindfulness meditation using the focus tools, you'll start to notice these visitors. As soon as you notice your attention has strayed from your anchor, name the visitor that you're greeting at that moment.

There's no reason to be angry or afraid of your visitors. It's best to be familiar with them so they don't surprise you later.

Here are some examples:

"I can't do this."	You're being visited by self-doubt
"My family will be so disappointed in me."	You're being visited by fear of failure
"I'm sure I got the last question wrong	You're being visited by the past
You start shaking	You're being visited by nervousness

So, how do you greet your visitors?

First, recognize who they are. Greet them by their names. It's not important that you come up with the perfect name or that you use the same type of name. Come up with a name that works for you, something that you can use to acknowledge to yourself that you have a familiar visitor.

If you prefer to give visitors proper names, go ahead. For example:

- Suzie Self-Doubt
- Mr. Alligator Anxiety
- Ms. Donut Distractions
- Mr. Sizzle Stressed Out

As you do this practice, you'll notice patterns and probably realize you have the same visitors over and over. That's common for most people.

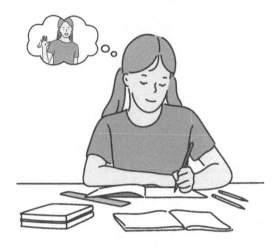

After you name them, acknowledge they're there. "Hi, Suzie Self-Doubt. I see you're here." After this acknowledgment, you can go back to your house and focus on your anchor. But some visitors stay a little longer. Simply greeting them isn't enough. For those, you have to sit with them. Eventually, they will go away. They don't live in your house. They're just passing through.

For visitors that are persistent and difficult, you can also use the tools from Chapter 9 on dealing with stress and difficult emotions.

1. *Get some challenging questions from a practice exam to work on. Set a timer. Try to feel the pressure of having to complete the questions in a limited amount of time, as you would in a test.*

2. *Start working on the questions.*

3. *When a distraction comes up, name and greet your visitor.*

4. *Go back to your questions.*

5. *Repeat steps two and three until your timer goes off.*

If you can practice this while you study, before test day, and become familiar with your visitors, it's more likely you won't have any emotional surprises during the test itself, which is the goal.

Go to the Mindfulness Toolbox now, and put a check mark next to the practices you've completed. Also, in the "Preferences/Notes" column, write down, "greet your visitors," if that's a practice you plan to use. Otherwise, just write down the first two tools. If you liked all three, it's fine to include all of them.

CHAPTER 7

STEP THREE — FIND RELAXATION

> "Almost everything will work again if you
> unplug it for a few minutes, including you."
>
> —ANNE LAMOTT

Relaxation is an important component of mindfulness. When you can relax your body, you open yourself to being able to focus. If you're too tense or wound up, it's harder to sit still and concentrate.

Realistically, though, you don't have time for a relaxing massage or yoga class before each study session, or while you're waiting for your test to start. Luckily, certain breathing tools can help quickly get your body and mind relaxed.

Start with Tool 1, and if it works, stick with it. If it doesn't work for you, or if you have the curiosity or time to check out more options, go on.

Tool 1: Box Breathing

This type of breathing has been demonstrated to calm your nervous system by creating even breathing. Even breathing creates a feedback loop with your brain, telling your brain that it can calm down.

- *Inhale slowly and deeply through your nose for a count of four, filling your lungs with air.*

- *Hold for a count of four. One, two, three, four.*

- *Exhale slowly through your mouth for a count of four, emptying your lungs completely.*

- *Hold for a count of four. One, two, three, four.*

- *Repeat.*

Continue for one to two minutes the first time you try this practice.

If that breathing tool relaxes you, stick with it. Box breathing can be your go-to relaxation technique. If not, move on to Tool 2.

Tool 2: Waterfall Breathing

Waterfall breathing is when your exhale is longer than your inhale. It's also called "5:7 breathing," to signify a five-count inhale, followed by a seven-count exhale. Don't get caught up in the name. The exact counts don't matter — what's important is that your exhale is longer than your inhale for the duration of this exercise. Your inhale stimulates your sympathetic nervous system (which is associated with action and energy), while your exhale stimulates your parasympathetic nervous system (which is associated with rest and digestion). By having a longer exhale than inhale, you stimulate your parasympathetic nervous system and invite your body to relax.

- *Inhale for five counts.*

- *Exhale for seven counts.*

- *Inhale — two – three – four – five.*

- *Exhale — two – three – four – five – six – seven.*

- *Repeat.*

Continue for one to two minutes the first time you do this practice.

If waterfall breathing works for you, stick with it. If you feel stressed out by just the thought and bother of counting your breaths, then go to Tool 3.

Tool 3: Belly Breathing

This may sound cliché, but deep breathing is very beneficial. A few deep breaths can change your body on a cellular level. When we're stressed out, our breathing can become shallow — quick inhales and exhales from the lungs. For many, this type of shallow breathing can become a normal pattern. Try this option to quickly relax your body by changing your breathing.

Keep one hand on your chest and the other hand on your belly, just below your rib cage.

Breathe in slowly and deeply through your nose, allowing your chest and lower belly to rise as you fill your lungs. Let your abdomen expand fully.

Now breathe out slowly through your mouth with your lips pursed.

Continue for five to ten deep breaths the first time you do this practice.

After you practice this a few times, you can do this without using your hands.

Relaxation—Choose and Implement

The relaxation tools in this section are not strictly mindfulness. Mindfulness is about being in touch with your natural breathing — however it is at the moment — and not controlling it. However, if your body is tense and rigid, it is hard to focus, which is the next step. So that's why relaxation is an important ingredient.

If you find it difficult to relax in one to two minutes, try practicing these exercises for longer periods of time. If you find your body still cannot relax, then do more extended relaxation practices: hot baths, yoga classes, massages. Relaxation is an important component of mindfulness for studying; it's difficult to focus when your body is tense.

Go to the Mindfulness Toolbox now and put a check mark next to the practices you've completed. Also, write down your preferred relaxation tool.

If you are short on time, proceed to Step 6 (Practice Your Tools and Create a Habit), which is in Chapter 10.

Everyone else, proceed to the next step, where you'll get to practice positive emotions. I'm sure you'll feel better after trying those out!

CHAPTER 8

STEP FOUR — CULTIVATE POSITIVE EMOTIONS

> "Sometimes your joy is the source of your smile, but sometimes your smile can be the source of your joy."
>
> — THICH NHAT HANH

Y ou are now on step four to learning mindfulness. This one will make you really happy.

It's common to think of meditation as something that helps you overcome the "bad things" in life, such as stress and negative emotions. It's true that meditation does that, but one of the overlooked benefits, which scientific research has uncovered, is that it can actually help you cultivate positive emotions, such as joy, happiness, and compassion.

By "practicing" these emotions with mindfulness, you actually strengthen the neural pathways of your brain that allow you to feel these emotions more often in your life, even outside meditation. That's one way mindfulness can actually make you a happier person.

So, let's get started and try cultivating positive emotions. For this step, try out all the tools. Then, pick out any you like to add to your toolbox.

Tool 1: Breathing and Smiling

Smiling is a quick way to connect with the positive. Research has found a connection between the muscles you use to smile and positive emotions. Yes, you smile when you're happy, but research shows that it works both ways: smiling can also cause you to feel good.

While researchers don't agree on the magnitude of the effect of a smile, this is one tool that's good to have in your arsenal. It's quick, easy, and can't do any harm.

Unlike simply smiling, this breathing and smiling practice brings awareness to your experience.

Thich Nhat Hanh, a world-famous meditation teacher, has dedicated his life to the practice of mindfulness, and this is one of his recommended practices.

Silently recite these lines as you breathe in and out and smile:

Breathing in, I calm body and mind.

Breathing out, I smile.

Dwelling in the present moment,

I know this is the only moment.

In this practice, smiling can help anchor you in both the present moment and positive emotions.

Tool 2: Self-Compassion

You probably wouldn't hesitate to send good thoughts and give a comforting hug to a friend in need. But how do you treat yourself when you're having a bad day? It's normal to be harsher on ourselves, judging and blaming ourselves when things are going badly.

If you were talking to a friend, you may say, "I'm sorry this is happening to you. That sounds so difficult. You're awesome, and I know you'll get through this."

But if something bad happens to you, you may think, "I'm such a failure. I'm so weak for feeling this way. My life sucks."

Self-compassion practices encourage a compassionate, kind attitude towards oneself. Easier said than done, for sure.

I have to admit, this topic is not very popular with students who are trying to study for an upcoming test.

"Self-compassion? What does that have to do with my SAT? I don't have time for this."

If you find the idea of these practices too "touchy-feely" or "hippy-dippy," you're not alone. Just remember that these have been proven to be effective mindfulness practices — and they're based in science.

Take a few deep breaths.

Close your eyes, if that feels comfortable for you.

Silently say two of the following phrases to yourself (pick whichever phrases feel right for you right now):

- *May I be happy*

- *May I be healthy*

- *May I be at ease*

- *May I be calm*

- *May I be safe*

- *May I be strong*

Give your full attention to each phrase.

Feel the intention of your wish for yourself as you say the phrase.

Leave enough silence between each one, so you can fully focus on each phrase before moving on to the next.

Repeat a few times. Take another breath, and open your eyes.

You can change the phrases to adapt them to what you feel you need in your life. Remember to choose positive phrases.

Tool 3: Gratitude

The inclusion of gratitude in a test prep book might stump you, but gratitude is actually an important mindfulness tool. Gratitude is one of many positive emotions you can practice and cultivate. It's about focusing on what's good in our lives and being thankful for the things we have, which counteracts stress and discontent.

Gratitude is about focusing on the good things in our life and expressing appreciation for what we have. It's taking a moment to notice and appreciate what we may take for granted — like having a roof over our heads, food, water, family, and maybe even friends.

To express gratitude, you can say things like: I am thankful, lucky, fortunate, humbled, or blessed.

Close your eyes, if that feels comfortable for you. Take a deep breath.

Think of three things in your life you're grateful for.

Say them silently to yourself:

I am grateful for _____ .

I am grateful for _____ .

I am grateful for _____ .

As you say each phrase to yourself, try to bring to mind an image of the person, animal, item, situation or quality — or whatever it is that you're grateful for.

Bring your attention fully to what you've named.

Notice if you feel any sense of thanks or gratitude.

If not, pause after that phrase and bring to mind why you feel grateful for that person, animal, or thing in your life. Why do you have appreciation? If you don't feel anything, that's fine. You don't need to force a feeling.

Move on to the next phrase. By just practicing repeating these lines, you're cultivating the seeds for gratitude. You may not feel it right away.

You can extend the gratitude practice above with the following:

Tool 3 Variation

In this tool, you send good wishes to another person. It's another way to rewire your brain with positive emotions.

Close your eyes, if that feels comfortable to you.

Think of a person in your life that you're grateful for. Imagine them in full detail: What they do look like? Sound like? Smell like? Do you know what they feel like?

Send some good wishes to this person by silently repeating the following phrases (or make up your own phrases):

- *May they be happy*
- *May they well*
- *May they live in ease*
- *May they be healthy*

Do this for one minute. Feel what sensations come up in your body as you think about this person/animal and as you send them these good wishes. What does it feel like?

Take a deep breath, and open your eyes if they were closed.

Positive emotions practices can be incorporated into your daily life. You can smile, express self-compassion, and appreciate people any time, not just while you're meditating. I encourage you to take these tools and put them into use throughout your day.

 What positive emotions practices worked well for you? Check them off in your Mindfulness Toolbox now.

CHAPTER 9

STEP FIVE – STRATEGIES FOR STRESS AND DIFFICULT EMOTIONS

> "Even in the midst of disturbance, the
> stillness of the mind can offer sanctuary."
>
> — STEPHEN RICHARDS

When my wrists suddenly stopped working in the middle of a busy college semester, I learned firsthand about the effects of bottled stress. On the outside, I didn't look or feel like I was overwhelmed. I didn't show outward signs of excessive stress — people knew me as a laid-back student from California. But stress had been building inside me, and it eventually found an outlet.

Whether you're the type of student who actively thinks, "I'm stressed out" most of the day, or someone who is too busy doing to even accommodate those thoughts, stress is possibly affecting you.

In addition to stress, you may be facing other strong or difficult emotions. It's normal for students, and everyone, to feel a range of emotions. It's a part of what it means to be human. If you don't allow yourself to feel these emotions, and instead suppress them or just let them simmer in the background, they may pop up when you least want to deal with them. Often, that may be while you're trying to prepare for a test.

The first two tools in this chapter provide ways you can confront stress and emotions in different ways:

1. In daily life: you can use the STOP tool when you feel challenged throughout your day. Sitting and closed eyes are not required!

2. In meditation practice: The RAIN tool can be used when stress or emotions come up during meditation practice. While sometimes you want to dismiss them as a distraction or a "visitor," it's useful to devote some sessions specifically to stay with emotions and address them.
The third tool, visualization, is helpful for general anxiety, or whenever you're worried about the future.

Try them all out, so you can have them handy when stress or emotions come up for you.

Tool 1: STOP

You can use this tool when faced with any stress or strong emotion that comes up during the day, even while studying or during a test.

Stop

Take a breath

Observe your body and mind

Proceed with mindfulness

In order to try out this tool, think of a mildly stressful situation you were recently in. Don't pick a highly stressful event because that will be difficult to use as you learn the tool. Just pick something that created a mild to moderate level of stress for you.

For example, maybe your history teacher gave you a pop quiz this week, and you weren't prepared. You should pick something that really happened to you. Then, follow these steps.

Close your eyes, if that feels comfortable for you. Visualize the situation completely. Where are you? Who are you with? What is happening? Imagine you're there right now. See if you can feel the emotions at the time something happened that triggered the emotions.

STOP: *As soon as you notice some signs of stress, pause. Stopping is not a long-term commitment. It could be only for a few seconds. But stop! Going forward while you're stressed out is not helping you.*

Take a breath: *This one's easy. Take a deep breath. Again, this only takes a few seconds.*

Observe: *Where in your body do you feel this? A heart beating fast, sweaty palms? Identify the place or places that are affected and observe what's happening for a few seconds. If you have time, also observe any thoughts you're having or any emotions that have come up for you.*

Proceed: *Go back to whatever you were doing, but this time more mindfully. You may even decide not to proceed and change your actions based on your check-in. There! A few seconds of your time, and hopefully you'll be more focused and relaxed going forward.*

Tool 2: RAIN

In Chapter 7, you learned how to deal with an emotion as a distraction or a visitor. Sometimes, however, an emotion will be so strong and dominant that it simply won't go away. It demands your attention, right then and there. In this case, when the emotion is hampering your ability to focus on your anchor, you need to direct your attention to the emotion itself.

The RAIN tool was first developed by mindfulness teacher, Michele McDonald. In this tool, your emotion itself becomes your anchor. You can use this tool when a strong emotion comes up during any of your mindfulness practices. If you're feeling a strong emotion, you can also start a meditation session with this tool. And if you just want to practice it in advance, try to visualize the situation. Visualization can bring up an emotion so you can feel it.

Follow these steps when an emotion arises:

Recognize: *Recognize that there's an emotion present for you right at the moment. This can be done by simply naming it.*

Allow: *Allow the emotion to be there, just as it is. This doesn't mean you're accepting the emotion permanently or liking the emotion, just that you're not fighting the fact that it's there. In other words, you give yourself permission to feel it.*

Investigate: *Investigate the physical sensations associated with the emotion. How do you know you're feeling it? Where do you feel it? What do you feel?*

Observe these sensations with awareness as you would observe your breath or another part of your body. Notice how the sensations may change as you observe them. If keeping your attention on the emotion becomes uncomfortable or feels overwhelming, change your focus to a neutral anchor — your breath, your body, or sounds. When you feel ready again, go back to your emotion. Repeat until you're done with the time you allocated for this practice.

Not Identifying: *You do not need to identify yourself with your emotion. An emotion is in you, but it does not define you. As you observed in your investigation, the sensations will change and eventually pass.*

My student Carlos found this practice helpful when he was overcome with nervousness a few days before an exam. He was trying to do a mindfulness focus practice, but the feeling of nervousness was so strong that he had trouble paying attention to his breath. So, instead, he decided to use RAIN. Here is how it worked for him:

R   Carlos **recognized** he was feeling the emotion of fear; he was fearful of an upcoming test.

A   Carlos **allowed** his mind and body to feel nervous instead of fighting it and scolding himself for feeling it.

I   Carlos observed that his heart was racing, his palms were sweating and his stomach had butterflies. As he **investigated** these sensations, he noticed they ebbed and flowed. He also noticed that his mind was full of thoughts about how difficult the test would be and how he thought he would fail it.

N   This is often the hardest step. It took several attempts with RAIN for Carlos to **not identify** the fear as part of himself. He had to get over the belief that fear would inevitably come up for him when he took a test.

Mindfulness teaches us to sit with emotions for increasingly longer lengths of time. When we do so, we don't have to force them out or ignore them. You'll find their power over you naturally diminishes with time.

Science supports this: According to Harvard brain scientist, Dr. Jill Bolte Taylor, an emotion's effect on your body lasts only up to ninety seconds, unless it's fueled by additional thoughts and narrative. This means, if you're able to sit with an emotion for ninety seconds, taking care not to think about the narrative surrounding an emotion (e.g., analyzing why you feel that way), the intensity and power of that emotion in your body will gradually fade and disappear in ninety seconds.

When you sit with emotions, it's also possible that you may confront underlying psychological conditions or issues you may be struggling with. If you suffer from emotions that seem overwhelming, or anything else that seems too challenging for you to handle on your own, ask a doctor, counselor, or other trusted adult to help you.

Tool 3: Visualization

While visualization is not strictly a mindfulness practice, it's a great tool to add to your toolbox, especially if you have experienced test-taking anxiety in the past.

Visualization means imagining something in your mind, the way you want it to happen, before it actually happens.

Here is a visualization you can start with. But you should feel free to customize it as needed.

1. *Take a few deep breaths.*

2. *Close your eyes, if that feels comfortable for you.*

3. *See yourself entering the room where you'll be taking the test. What does it look like?*

4. *Imagine feeling calm, confident, and at ease. What does that feel like?*

5. *See yourself sitting down at the desk or table where you'll be taking the exam.*

6. *Imagine feeling calm, confident, and at ease. What does that feel like?*

7. *See yourself receiving the test from your instructor. See yourself going through the test and answering each question with confidence and ease.*

8. *Take a few deep breaths.*

9. *Experience the feeling of confidence that comes from knowing that you're selecting the right answers. Envision completing the test within the time limit, still feeling the satisfaction and confidence that comes with a job well done.*

10. *Finally, visualize yourself completing the test and handing it in or clicking submit.*

11. *Take a few more deep breaths.*

As you practice visualizations, keep these three things in mind:

1. *Keep your visualizations as realistic and detailed as possible.*

2. *Remember to stay aware of your breathing.*

3. *Practice what you're feeling: calm, at ease and confident. As much as you can, practice conjuring up the state of mind/ emotion that you want to be feeling during the test.*

Your Mindfulness Toolbox is filling up! Check off the practices you've completed in your Mindfulness Toolbox. If you have any preferred tools, write that down, too. Now it's time to practice all these tools, which you'll get to do in the next chapter where you'll complete the final step in learning mindfulness.

CHAPTER 10

STEP SIX — JUMP START YOUR MINDFULNESS PRACTICE IN TWO WEEKS ... OR TWO DAYS

> "Motivation is what gets you started.
> Habit is what keeps you going."
>
> —JIM RYUN

Congratulations, you've made it to the last step of learning mindfulness. Check out your Mindfulness Toolbox. By now, you've filled it with many useful tools, but to be effective, these tools need to be practiced. The more you practice, the more effective they'll be for you.

This last step is probably the most important of them all.

As I stated earlier in this book, mindfulness is not a magic pill you can pop into your mouth and forget. Like any worthwhile goal, some effort is required.

That's why your goal in this chapter is to create a daily habit. The most effective way to do this is with small, incremental steps every day.

You can start your mindfulness habit in just two weeks of daily practice. Taking a few minutes each day for fourteen days is a manageable goal!

After you've set a daily mindfulness habit in motion, you're ready to integrate mindfulness fully with your studying and test-taking, which we will cover in Part III. But even before you formally combine mindfulness with studying, you may start noticing the benefits in your studying right away: you're likely to be more focused and less anxious.

If you are really short of time, you can practice these tools in an intense two-day period, which is covered at the end of this chapter. However, keep this as a last resort. You'll likely get better results and enjoy the process more if you practice gradually over the course of two weeks.

Pick Your Time of Day

For the next two weeks, find a time of day where you think you'll have minimal distractions.

Everyone has their own schedules and preferences. When do you think you can most easily squeeze in fifteen minutes? Many people prefer to do this as soon as they wake up in the morning or right before bed, but there is no right or wrong time of day.

Take action now, and commit to a time. Complete the sentence below:

For the next two weeks, I will make an effort to meditate (from two minutes to fifteen minutes) during the following time of day: _____ .

Of course, some days it may be difficult for you to meditate at the chosen time, and that's okay. If you know you have a game or weekend event that conflicts with your usual time, just reschedule your meditation — move it to another time of the day that will work.

Remember, it will only a few minutes each day; you're not making a major time commitment.

Start Now

Don't wait for a perfect two weeks in the future where your calendar is free. That's not going to happen. Commit to starting today (or tomorrow if your time of day has already passed). When you put things off, you increase the likelihood they won't happen.

Make it Non-Negotiable

What does non-negotiable mean? It means you do it no matter what; no matter how sleepy or tired or busy you are.

My student Lynn was determined to start meditating, but she told me about the obstacles she was facing. "I started out full of motivation. The first two days were great. Then, I had a dinner the next day and got home late, so I was too tired. The next day, I had a big school project due. And then I had a game that went on until 9 p.m., and I had to come home and do my homework after. Suddenly, I had missed three days, and I felt too discouraged. I just gave up."

Lynn's experience is normal, especially for overscheduled, busy students. It can be hard to find even a few minutes a day to commit to something new.

To help overcome this challenge, make meditation a non-negotiable activity.

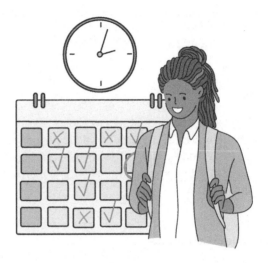

What does non-negotiable mean? It means you do it no matter what; no matter how sleepy or tired or busy you are. It's like brushing your teeth. It's not something most people will skip, no matter what.

Tell yourself it's only for fourteen days. When I first attempted to make meditation a daily habit, I wouldn't let myself go to sleep without meditating, period. No matter how tired I was. No matter how enticing and warm and comfy my bed looked.

Once you complete the initial two weeks, you'll likely start feeling tangible benefits in your own life. Often, that will supply you with the motivation to continue.

Don't Give Up if You Miss a Day

Despite making it non-negotiable, you may still miss a day. Life happens, and that's okay.

Part of mindfulness is being kind and compassionate to yourself, so don't beat yourself up over a missed day or two.

If this happens, don't get discouraged and give up. Just jump right back where you left off! You are aiming for fourteen days in a row, but if you miss a couple of days along the way, don't let that derail you.

Practical Details to Start Your Mindfulness Habit

How many minutes do you need?

While science doesn't provide an exact answer as to how many minutes you need to obtain the benefits of mindfulness, many researchers suggest that fifteen to twenty minutes a day of mindfulness meditation can yield measurable results.

For the two-week plan in this chapter, build up to fifteen minutes gradually. Follow this schedule:

Day	Number of Minutes
Day 1–Day 2	2 Minutes
Day 3–Day 6	5 Minutes
Day 7–Day 10	10 Minutes
Day 11–Day 14	15 Minutes

If you find increasing the number of minutes to be difficult, be patient with yourself. Try your best. If it just feels too challenging, stay with a lower number of minutes. It's more important that you meditate consistently than aim for too long and end up abandoning the effort.

If the time seems to fly by for you and your schedule allows, you can increase your meditation time to twenty minutes. But that's optional.

What exactly do I do with all those minutes?

Okay, you've settled on a time of day and made meditation non-negotiable for a certain number of minutes. So, what exactly do you do with those minutes? If you followed the steps in the previous chapters, you've already learned everything you need to know to start your meditation practice. Let's refresh your memory and recall some of your preferred tools here:

Step 1   My preferred focus practice is _____.

Step 2   My preferred tool for dealing with distractions is _____.

Step 3   My preferred tool for relaxing is _____.

Step 4   My preferred tool for cultivating positive emotions is _____.

Step 5   My preferred tool for managing stress and difficult emotions
               is _____.

I recommend always starting with a minute of a relaxation tool. This helps calm your nervous system and put your body more at ease for the rest of the meditation. Below are guidelines to fill your time, but you're free to customize your practice with whatever mindfulness practice you feel is most helpful. Remember, the key is simply to practice mindfulness for the allotted time each day.

Suggested Practices

For the first six days (Days 1–6), keep it simple. Start each session with one minute of relaxation and then continue for the rest of your scheduled time with focus. If distractions or stress come up for you, use those tools as needed.

For the remaining days (Days 7–14), repeat what you did in week one for the first five minutes, or as long as you are comfortably able. Then, use the remaining time to practice other tools from Part II.

Use a timer to set your time period before you start your session. If you have a kitchen timer or stopwatch, it's better to use than a cell phone because you'll minimize the distraction of having your phone nearby. But if you don't have these, you can use your phone timer.

If you find it's hard to do this by yourself, it is fine to use guided meditations to fill your time, too. You can check out www.MindOverScatterBook.com/audio for guided meditations from this book or use any other guided mindfulness meditation you find helpful.

What happens after two weeks?

If you've followed the steps in this chapter, you're probably already experiencing some of the benefits of mindfulness. The results may not be immediate and sensational — there are no firecrackers and drumrolls to signify accomplishment and success. Still, you may start to notice small moments where you feel calmer, less anxious, and more in control of your mind.

"You may start to notice small moments where you feel calmer, less anxious, and more in control of your mind."

Your goal in reading this book is to use mindfulness to become a better test-taker, so after two weeks of practice, it's time to start integrating mindfulness into your studying and test-taking. You will continue a daily habit, but now tie it with test-taking.

If you feel you need more practice with mindfulness tools or are enjoying the daily routine, keep going with your daily practice, even outside test-taking! The benefits to you will keep increasing, even after two weeks.

Two-Day Jump Start

If you don't have two weeks to practice mindfulness tools, and you need to jump in and use these tools for test-taking, then read this section.

Set aside two days where you don't have too many scheduled events. A weekend would be ideal, but you can adapt this even for school days. Create seven practice sessions a day. Start each hour, or every other hour, with a few minutes of mindfulness, gradually increasing your practice time. You can adapt this schedule to make time for school or other scheduled events.

Sample daily schedule

8 a.m.	2 minutes
10 a.m.	5 minutes
Noon	5 minutes
2 p.m.	10 minutes
4 p.m.	10 minutes
6 p.m.	15 minutes
8 p.m.	15 minutes

What should you do with those minutes? Use the "Suggested Practices" section above for ideas — but remember, creating scheduled times and sticking with them is more important than the particular practices you choose.

Overcoming Challenges

Ten or fifteen minutes is too long

If the time period feels too long and you're restless and bored, try changing your focus to your restlessness and boredom. How do you know that you're restless or bored? What does that feel like? Do you feel uncomfortable with staying still? Do you desperately want to check your phone for messages? What does that feel like?

Mindfulness, at its core, is paying attention to what's happening in the present moment with openness and curiosity. Try experimenting with an attitude of curiosity as you bring your attention to whatever it is that you're feeling right now.

If you've tried all this, and the allotted time is still too long for you, don't worry. You can also try going back to the previous time increment (two minutes or five minutes) and stay there for more days. In this way, you can increase your time more gradually. If you cannot get to fifteen minutes in two weeks, that's okay. You'll still get benefits, even if you limit your practice to a shorter time each day.

You're not sure what you're supposed to be doing

If you're feeling confused about what you're supposed to be doing, you might be trying too hard to do the "right" thing. Your only instruction is to try to pay attention to the present moment. If you can't do this, that's okay — just bring yourself back to your breath, your body, or the sounds around you, as soon as you notice you're lost in thought. That's how you learn mindfulness and grow your mindfulness muscle.

If you feel you need more specific guidance during your allotted time, you're not alone. A lot of people feel that way. It doesn't mean you can't benefit from meditation. Start by reading the prompts in the previous chapters. Close your eyes and give it a go. Guided meditation also can be helpful if you feel lost.

Meditating makes you sleepy

Usually, when you close your eyes, you're preparing to sleep, so it is not surprising that many of us get sleepy when we try to meditate. If this happens to you, try one of these options:

1. **Open your eyes.** It's fine to practice mindfulness with your eyes open; it just can be a little more difficult because you'll notice more distractions. When your eyes are open, be sure to keep your gaze downward.

2. **Stand up.** This can help you wake up. You can keep practicing mindfulness even as you stand. You may need to open your eyes to keep your balance.

3. **Walk.** Open your eyes, stand up, and slowly start to walk. As you walk, shift your focus to the sensations in your body. Pay attention to your feet and other parts of your body. When you feel alert, sit down again and resume your earlier practice.

Meditating is causing you pain

If sitting down for the allotted time is painful, try changing your posture. You can move from the floor to a chair or vice versa. You can also try the movement suggestions in the "Meditating makes you sleepy" section above.

While you want to be comfortable during meditation, it's also good not to change postures so much that it's a distraction. If you feel initial pain that seems bearable, you can investigate that pain using the tools of mindfulness. Go back to Chapter 9 and practice the tools there.

Other challenges

Other challenges may come up for you. Mindfulness is simple but not necessarily easy. Give yourself some love and some patience and use creative thinking to solve the issues rather than giving up. You can do it!

What You've Learned

✔ Schedule your meditation time.

✔ Make daily practice non-negotiable.

✔ If you fall off track, get right back on.

✔ Gradually add time to your daily practice of fifteen minutes. If you feel like you can handle more time, go up to twenty minutes.

✔ Start each session with relaxation, and then try a mix of other mindfulness practices.

PART III

MINDFULNESS FOR STUDYING AND TEST-TAKING

CHAPTER 11

HOW TO BE A HAPPY TEST-TAKER — FINDING JOY AND PURPOSE

> *"The secret of happiness is not in doing what one likes, but in liking what one does."*
>
> —JAMES M. BARRIE

Take a deep breath. You've now learned and practiced mindfulness tools, which have the potential to help you score better. It's time to apply it all to test-taking. This is where the magic happens. In the next three chapters, you'll learn specific methods to integrate mindfulness into your studying and test-taking.

So what's happiness got to do with it?

The whole point of learning mindfulness is to find a different approach to the "grit your teeth and get through it" approach to test-taking.

The same tools that can boost your test score can also help you be happier as you do so.

Before we get into the details of how to apply mindfulness tools to studying and test-taking (which is coming up in the following chapters), let's figure out how you can enjoy the process.

In Chapter 3, we learned that your happiness is more linked to how much attention you're paying to the present, rather than what you're doing. You can be unhappy in Disneyland or any other place where you find would normally be happy. The opposite is also true: you can be happy washing dishes — a task you don't usually associate with a source of joy.

If you're like most students, you don't usually jump for joy at the prospect of studying and taking a test. But you can learn to cultivate happiness even during these tasks, no matter how much you think you hate them.

An Alternative to Negative Thinking and Escapism from Studying

Do any of these thoughts sound familiar to you?

> "I hate studying."
> "This is so boring."
> "This is so hard."
> "I want this to be over."
> "I wish I could be with my friends right now."
> "I really want to check my phone."

If you have these thoughts in your head while you're studying, you're not studying effectively. Your mind is occupied and full of negativity instead of paying attention to the present moment.

It's common to want to escape experiences we feel negative about. So, if you're trying to avoid feeling bad while studying, you may try to escape by:

- Eating/snacking on sugary treats.
- Constantly checking on text messages and other notifications on your phone.
- Having the TV on.

Nothing is wrong with you for doing this. It's normal and common. By engaging in these pleasant activities at the same time as studying, you can distract yourself from the perceived pain of studying.

But the problem is: these distractions don't solve the problem of your dislike of studying, and they don't make you any happier in the long run.

The mindfulness approach is that, instead of escaping the pain of the experience, you immerse yourself fully in it. You make studying itself your anchor. When negative thoughts arise as you're studying, recognize them as distractions and label them as "thoughts" and go back to the present moment experience of studying.

How to Be Fully Present While Studying

Even if you don't like washing dishes, you can find happiness in the task if you change your object of focus. Instead of thinking about how annoying washing dishes is, you can direct your attention to immerse yourself fully in the experience: notice the feeling of soapy bubbles against skin, the warmth of the running water, the rainbow of colors in your dishware.

If you pay complete attention to your task — what do you actually experience while studying?

In Chapter 5, you practiced directing your focus to different anchors such as your breath, your body, or sounds.

Now, it's time to put your mindfulness tools to use and make studying itself your anchor of attention.

If it feels silly or counterintuitive to immerse yourself in an activity you think of as unpleasant, just remind yourself of the science. Science shows that if you fully pay attention to what you're doing — even studying — you may find happiness while doing the task!

Alien Study Discovery Tour

Here's a fun activity that can help you understand what it feels like to immerse yourself in studying.

Pretend you're an alien on earth for the first time and experience this thing called "studying." Approach studying like you've never done it before. Each time you study, open up a book or open up your laptop with a sense of adventure and newness.

To do this, avoid just simply falling back into your old habits and routines. Don't mindlessly open up your study materials, as you're likely then to fall into the same habits that may not have been so helpful before.

Start with an attitude of adventure and curiosity. Ready?

Get out your study materials now, but don't open any books or devices yet.

Pretend this is all new for you. You get to study today as if for the very first time. Now, pick up those materials and examine them with all five senses.

- *What do you see? What are the colors and shapes of your study materials and study space? What else is in your view and surroundings?*

- *What do you hear? Is there music, voices, or the dull hum of appliances around?*

- *What do you taste? You don't have to have anything in your mouth for this, just notice any tastes — or no taste — on your tongue in the moment.*

- *What sensations of touch are you feeling? Notice the touch of the pencil against your fingers. Feel the hardness of the laptop as you type into it. Pay attention to the tingling in your fingers as your press the keyboard. Notice the pressure of a book against your lap and the heat emanating from your laptop.*

> • *What are you smelling? Do the paper or the devices have any smells? Bring them to your nose and take a sniff.*

After you've completed this five senses exploration, off you go! Start studying. Be curious about what you are studying now, whether it's math or science or vocabulary. Be really curious. How interesting! How lucky you get to learn this! This is secret stuff; you may even bring it back to your home planet after. Delight in it!

When you find yourself bored or distracted while studying, go back to your curiosity about your present moment experience. Briefly check in again with your senses. Then, return to studying. You may feel silly doing this, but remember that, if you bring your full attention to a task — with an attitude of openness, curiosity, and kindness — you're more likely to find happiness in it.

Be Happy by Anchoring in Studying

If playing make believe isn't for you, there's also a more straightforward way to fully immerse yourself in the studying experience.

Here are three things you can focus on while studying to keep you present:

1. **The content** — the subject matter of what you are reading, memorizing or doing.
2. **Tangible items associated with studying** — your writing utensils, devices, books, and study space.
3. **Your body** — the sensations that are happening in your body while studying.

While your ultimate goal is to focus on the specific content you're studying, that can be hard to do. It's inevitable that you'll be distracted and be interrupted by thoughts. The subject matter you're studying requires mental effort, sometimes difficult and sustained work. It's tiring. Your mind needs a break and will want to escape.

Instead of letting your mind be distracted (which also causes unhappiness), redirect your attention to the physical experiences and sensations of studying (the tangible items and any feelings in your body).

Try this practice and see if you can find some joy even while studying.

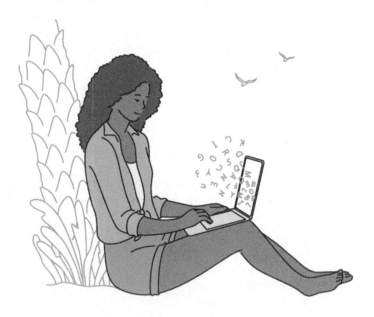

 Locate study materials that you need to focus on and absorb. Whether it's in the form of a book or on your laptop, get it out.

1. *Take a few moments to physically connect with the object you have in front of you, whether it's a book or device. Notice what it looks like. What color is it? Is it shiny or dull? Take note of its texture. What does it feel like when you touch it? Do you notice that it's soft or hard? Is it smooth or rough?*

2. *Start studying, and keep at it until you notice your mind wanders.*

3. *When you notice your mind has wandered, bring your attention back to the physical object in front of you or what you're touching.*

4. *Then, bring your awareness to the sensations of the experience itself. What does it feel like to study? What do your eyes feel like when you're studying? Do they feel strained or sore or tired? What do the keys feel like beneath your fingers? What sensations do you notice as you touch the keyboard? Do you feel the pressure of the laptop? The hardness of the keys? The smoothness of your mouse? Do you feel the crispness of paper? The smell of a new book?*

5. *Return to studying. When your mind wanders again, repeat.*

To be clear, your aim is not to replace focus on the subject matter. It's only when your mind wanders from the studying that you should go back to the sensations of your study materials and your body as a way to anchor yourself back into the present moment.

Gratitude Is Happiness

In Chapter 8 you practiced cultivating gratitude. If you're in the throes of pain just thinking about an upcoming test, it might seem unimaginable to muster gratitude in your life right now.

But see if you can find some gratitude — without forcing it — for being able to take the test at all. As fearsome as it may seem, taking the test does potentially open up doors for you. Maybe you have the opportunity to get an A in a class and improve your GPA, improve your chances of admissions to your top choice school, or feel the satisfaction of accomplishing a goal. Realize that not everyone even has the ability to take the tests you have access to.

Are there any people in your life that are supporting you or making it possible for you to take the test? Maybe you have the support of your family, a counselor, a teacher, or a friend.

Do the gratitude practices in Chapter 8, thinking of what you're grateful that relates to the specific test that is coming up. Think of a person who is supporting you as you study for this test.

While expressing appreciation may seem unrelated to your test, remind yourself that serious scientific studies have validated gratitude practices.

Find a Purpose to Motivate Yourself

As you use mindfulness to boost your test scores and your GPA, keep in mind your ultimate purpose. Why do you want to ace that test? Is it because it will increase your chances of getting a scholarship to help you afford your education? Is it to prove to yourself that you can do it? Do you want to get into medical school so you can become a doctor? Is this the first step to getting into a good MBA program and becoming financially successful? Or perhaps you haven't given it much thought at all — you want to score high because everyone else seems to want that.

There's no right answer about why you want to do well on your tests, and there's no need to judge yourself based on why you have this goal. But if you can uncover your true purpose and be clear on it, it can help motivate you as well as put the outcome of your test in perspective. Luckily, mindfulness is more than a productivity tool for high performance. You can use the time and space it creates for deeper reflection on your purpose and meaning.

Take a deep breath.

Ask yourself: What motivates you? Why do you want to do well on this test?

Tap into this source of purpose and meaning while you're studying.

What You've Learned

✔ You can find happiness in studying if you're fully present.

✔ Approach studying with curiosity and activate all your senses.

✔ Bring gratitude to your test-taking.

✔ Uncover your purpose to bring meaning and motivation to studying.

CHAPTER 12

THREE LETTERS THAT WILL CHANGE THE WAY YOU STUDY FOR TESTS

> "Start where you are. Use what you have. Do what you can."
>
> —ARTHUR ASHE

So far, you've learned and practiced the tools of mindfulness, and you've discovered how to bring curiosity, and even joy, into the act of studying.

Now, the question is: How do you use these tactics to study mindfully and boost your test scores?

Why You Should Use Mindfulness While You Study

My student Jasmine was so excited when she was able to work up to fifteen minutes of daily meditation. But when it came closer to the test, she panicked and stopped practicing.

"I don't have time for this now. I have to study! I'm so behind."

Suddenly, the fifteen minutes that seemed like nothing at all a few weeks ago feels like too long to spend on anything but studying. Time becomes a precious resource as a test draws near, and it's easy to abandon practices, even when we logically know they can help us.

You may think, "In those ten minutes, I can learn more vocabulary words."

Imagine you're sitting down to study. You probably carved out just enough time in your schedule to do it. You don't want to take time out to meditate because it sounds counterintuitive to do something other than spending time learning, memorizing, and practicing the subjects that you will be tested on. But remember: research shows that mindfulness will improve your mental performance. So, what I'm going to show you now is how to incorporate mindfulness into your studying.

Learn the Three Step Process of RFI

Three letters you need to remember to boost your studying and test-taking are RFI. This stands for Relax, Focus, and Intent.

Before you start studying or doing your homework, spend a few minutes doing the following:

Relax	Do a relaxation practice using one of the tools (See Chapter 7) for one minute.
Focus	Do a focus practice (See Chapter 5) using your breath, body, or sounds. Do this for three minutes.
Intent	Set a clear intent as to what you want to accomplish during your study session.

Your intent should be as specific as possible. For example, "In the next twenty-five minutes, I will go over the math section of my practice exam for my ACT and review all the questions I got wrong."

You can say this out loud or in your mind, but make sure it is a clear and specific statement. Be realistic when you create your intent — create a task you can do in the time you have.

Three letters you need to remember to boost your studying and test-taking are RFI. This stands for Relax, Focus, and Intent.

Now, open your eyes if they are closed. Your body should be relaxed, alert, and focused.

Let your task be your anchor now. Instead of paying attention to your body, breath, or sounds, direct all your attention to studying, doing homework, completing a practice exam, or whatever task it was you stated in your intent.

When you get distracted from your studying (or your task), as soon as you realize your mind has wandered, gently direct your attention back to your task. The task you set out to accomplish in your intention is now your anchor.

By using RFI, you actually transform your regular studying time to mindfulness practice time. You're just changing the focus of your meditation to the subject you're studying.

 Try this now. Get out your study materials. Find a task that should take you about five minutes. Go through the RFI steps above and see if you can move your anchor from your breath/ body/sounds to what you're studying.

Here's an example of Connor using RFI to study for an upcoming test.

Relax	Connor sits at his desk, where he usually studies. He closes his eyes and spends one minute doing box breathing. Breathing in for four counts, holding for four counts, breathing out for four counts and holding for four counts. He does this for one minute.
Focus	Next, Connor brings his attention to his preferred anchor, his breath. He notices his stomach expanding and contracting with each breath. He gets distracted and starts thinking about what he's going to eat for dinner. As soon as he notices that he's distracted, Connor uses the labeling thoughts tool (Chapter 6). Connor returns his focus to his breath.
Intent	Connor states to himself, "In the next twenty-five minutes, I'm going to complete all the practice questions in my study guide and go over the answers."

Connor opens his eyes and starts doing his practice questions. He successfully keeps his attention on them for a while, but then, he starts thinking about an upcoming baseball game. As soon as he realizes he's been distracted, he makes a mental note to himself, "There's a thought." He gently brings his attention back to his practice questions.

Get Better at RFI

When you first start using RFI, you may find it challenging to stay focused on your studying for long periods of time. That's okay. Start with short study tasks — five to ten minutes. Build up to twenty-five minutes.

It's normal and totally acceptable not to be able to stay completely focused for the entire study time. So, as soon as you notice you're distracted, use the tools you learned in Part II to gently bring your attention back to your studying. By doing this over and over again, you'll start to improve your mindfulness muscles, even while studying.

After you gain practice in RFI, you can experiment with changing the number of minutes for each part of the relaxation, focus and intent practices, depending on what works best for you.

The Foolproof Way to Study Using RFI

After you've tried RFI a few times to begin a study session, you're ready to create blocks of study time using mindfulness. Follow these steps:

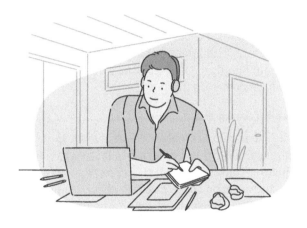

Step 1. Break your study time into blocks.

Each block should be twenty-five minutes. If you feel that's too long for you to stay focused, you can reduce it to twenty minutes. If you can stay focused longer, increase it to thirty minutes.

The process of breaking up study time into short, focused intervals, followed by a break, is called the Pomodoro Technique. This method is compatible with the mindfulness practice because the emphasis is on creating a concentrated period of time where you know you need to focus. It's short enough that you can realistically focus for that period of time, and you know you have a break coming.

To be most effective, minimize your distractions, including your notifications. During the study block, you're making a commitment to study and not do anything else.

Step 2. Start each study block with RFI.

Relax for one minute, focus for three minutes, and then spend one minute setting your intent.

Step 3. Study with mindfulness.

For the duration of your study block, use your study material as your anchor of focus. Every time you find yourself distracted, bored, restless, or anything else, just gently bring your attention back to your studying and use your Mindfulness Toolbox to help you deal with whatever comes up.

Step 4: Take a break.

Take a five-minute break. Set a timer to make sure you stay on schedule. Go outside, get a snack, stretch, move, or do whatever you feel like to rest. To keep yourself focused, it's best not to get on social media or check e-mail during this time, as those can pull you away from the studying task.

Step 5: Repeat.

It's now time to start RFI and your twenty-five-minute study block again. You can continue for three or four study blocks. At that point, take a longer break or stop studying for the day.

If you don't have time to do another study block, that's fine. It's always okay to just do one study block if that's all you have time for.

Following these steps to break up your study time into blocks can create a "container," where you feel safe and focused while studying.

Scheduling Mindfulness

Now that you know how to do a mindful study block, it's time to make sure it happens. Open up your calendar and literally schedule in blocks. Just as you would respect other events and classes in your schedule, commit to set times for studying for your test.

As soon as you know you have a test coming up, start adding study blocks (devoted to that test) into your schedule. Otherwise, it's too easy to get caught up with homework and last-minute projects.

This is particularly important if you have a big test coming up, like the ACT, SAT, GRE, LSAT, or MCAT. It's important to plan in advance and schedule time for taking practice exams and studying in regular intervals prior to the test.

Add study blocks into your calendar now. Where can you fit in three or four study blocks in a row? Where can you squeeze in just one? In your calendar entry, note what test you're studying for. Now you have to respect your commitment. If you absolutely cannot make it when the time comes up, reschedule it on your calendar right then — no waiting for later to reschedule.

Use a Study Buddy to Keep Yourself on Track

For some students, it can be helpful to have someone to share a study block with. You can share a timer and keep each other on track. Just make sure your study buddy is equally committed to creating a distraction-free environment where you can study. Feel free to walk them through RFI (sometimes teaching it to others can be the best way to master a concept yourself), or they can skip that part and just join you for the focused study time. You can share a study space, or even do this on Zoom or a virtual platform.

It's also possible that having another person around while studying can be distracting. So, like so much of mindfulness, experiment and see what works best for you.

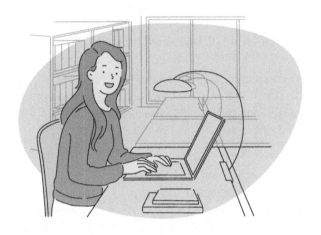

Keep Up Your Daily Habit

In Chapter 10, you built up your mindfulness muscle by practicing daily for fourteen days (or two days if you were short on time).

And now you've learned how to practice mindfulness while studying, so you can easily get your daily practice minutes in without having to find extra time in the day.

Try to keep the momentum of your initial fourteen-day (or two-day) practice, and keep mindfulness as a daily habit. Make sure you practice mindfulness for a few minutes before each study session or test.

If your total mindfulness minutes on any day add up to less than fifteen (or twenty, if that was your goal), schedule a few extra minutes of mindfulness at the end of the day.

Or, if you're the type of person who prefers to have a regular time and place for your mindfulness practice, keep doing what you did during the first two weeks. Meditate at the same time for fifteen or twenty minutes, and make it non-negotiable.

If you need extra motivation, review the studies in Chapter 3 again. Remember the beneficial effects are cumulative — the more you practice, the more advantages you will yield. Stress levels can be reduced, and your brain can actually change in just eight weeks. So keep on going!

What You've Learned

The best way to implement mindfulness when you're studying is to:

✔ Follow the RFI steps: Relax, Focus, Intent.

✔ Practice mindful studying for five-minute sessions, gradually increasing to twenty-five minutes.

✔ Create study blocks and start each one with RFI.

✔ Schedule mindfulness into your calendar.

✔ Consider finding a study buddy.

✔ Keep building a mindfulness habit.

CHAPTER 13

MINDFULNESS FOR TEST DAY

By now, you've put mindfulness practices to use when studying for a test, but don't forget that you can also use mindfulness to successfully navigate the test itself.

Use RFI for Test-Taking

By test day, you should have plenty of practice using RFI for studying.

Experiment and customize

One of the most important things you can do before a test is take as many practice exams as time allows. When you take the practice exams, keep the conditions as close to actual test day as possible. Be in a quiet space, turn off all notifications, and use a timer to limit yourself to the permitted test time.

Use RFI before each practice test. Then, try the same RFI techniques you used for studying and adapt them for test-taking. You can do that by experimenting with different lengths of relaxation practice, different lengths of focus practice, and different intents. Often, you may find you want to spend a longer time with relaxation right before a test and shorten the time for focus. You also want to try setting intentions specific to taking a certain test.

For example, you can try this one adaptation of RFI and see if it works for you. Remember, it may change from test to test, which is why it's important to try the technique during practice exams.

Relax	2 minutes
Focus	1 minute
Intent	30 seconds

At the end of RFI, direct all your focus to the test. Just as when you were studying, if distractions come up, label the thought or emotion or acknowledge the visitor, and gently direct yourself back to the test.

Set the right intent

Make sure you practice the exact intent you want to use during the test beforehand. You may want to set an intent about how you want to be when taking the test.

"I will be relaxed and focused during this test."

Or, if you want to focus on the outcome, your intent can be: "I will answer all the questions correctly and ace this test." You may find that an outcome-focused intent will create pressure for you, or it might help motivate you. The point is that, during the practice exams, you can try out different intents and see what works for you.

Figure out when you'll do RFI

Make sure you engage in RFI before the test gets handed out. Don't use up your actual test time.

Also, consider your circumstances. If you can't realistically do RFI, or you feel too self-conscious for whatever reason (although no one has to know), you can do it in the car or before you enter the room.

You may also settle for a shorter version of RFI — a few relaxation breathes, a few focused breaths and intent.

Handle stress and difficult emotions

By now, you know that when thoughts or emotions arise while trying to focus, you can simply label them and direct your attention back to your anchor — whether that is your breath or study materials.

But for bigger issues that can't be so easily dismissed, the underlying stresses and larger emotions, labeling may not be enough. They will poke their heads up and stay with you during your test — potentially disrupting your performance.

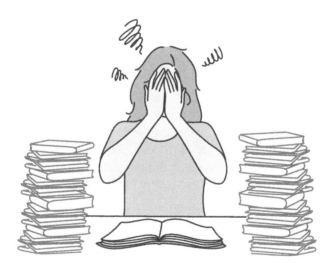

There's a way to deal with these during longer mindfulness sessions, as we've explored in Chapter 9, but this isn't something you'll have time for during the test. If this is likely to come up for you, do the following exercise before test day.

1. Take out a piece of paper or open a blank document. Set a timer for five minutes and write down a list of everything stressful in your life. Don't censor yourself. Just write anything and everything.

2. Number your list.

3. Go through each issue in order and try the practices in Chapter 9. You don't have to tackle every issue during the same meditation session — spread them out over as many days as you have until the test.

4. If anything seems too difficult or overwhelming for you to handle, speak to a trusted adult or professional counselor.

Test Anxiety

One of my students, Amelia, used to freeze when she read an exam question she didn't know the answer to. Like a deer in headlights, she couldn't think or act. At first, she said this never happened during practice exams.

However, after Amelia started a mindfulness practice and became more aware of what was going on in her mind, she noticed that she did experience stress and a sense of distraction when confronted with a question she didn't know the answer to even during practice exams. While it wasn't the same intensity as the freezing she experienced during an actual test, she used the opportunity to try out mindfulness tools.

If you've experienced test anxiety right before or during a test, spend some time before the test creating a strategy to deal with it. Anxiety may come in the form of panic, freezing, or jitters.

Practice tests often don't incite the same anxiety that a real test can bring, but it's still helpful to practice options for dealing with anxiety in advance.

You can try these three options:

- **Visualization.** When you repeatedly imagine yourself taking a test with ease, it's easier to do it on the real day. Do the visualization practice in Chapter 9 as often as possible. Try adding a visualization to your RFI. When you get to Intent, imagine yourself taking the test relaxed, calm, and at ease.
- **Focus on a neutral part of your body.** By neutral, I mean a place that doesn't feel painful or affected by the anxiety. You probably don't want to focus on your heart, for example, as it may be racing. For many students, it's helpful to direct their attention to their feet. You can practice this by doing the focus practices in Chapter 5.
- **Belly breathing before and during the test.** You can try taking a deep breath every time you turn a page or go to a new section. Belly breathing is described in more detail in Chapter 7.
- **Observe what is happening in your body.** Is it a fast breath, sweaty palms, rapid heart rate, or something else? Use the STOP technique from Chapter 9. Note that this is the opposite of the second bullet point above. It may be overwhelming for you to observe the anxiety itself, in which case, focusing on a neutral body part may work best. Try both out.

Take lots of practice tests and experiment with what works best for you to do before and during the test. What works for you may not be the same as what works for someone else.

The Day Before the Test

The day before the test is an important one. Studying and cramming on the last day won't be helpful. You don't want to stress yourself out or get tired on this day.

This is the day to calmly review your notes, prepare yourself mentally for the test, and take care of yourself physically. Make sure you eat healthy meals and get to sleep on time.

The day before the test, try this mindfulness routine:

RFI before reviewing your notes (Chapter 12)	5 minutes
Visualization practice (Chapter 9)	2 minutes
Positive emotions practice (Chapter 8)	2 minutes
Longer mindfulness meditation session in the evening, including relaxation and focus practices (Chapters 5 and 7)	10 to 20 minutes

The Day of the Test

The big day is here! Test day. Take a deep breath. Stay calm and relaxed. Eat healthy meals. You will do the best you can do.

Starting in the morning, do relaxation practices for a few minutes. No one needs to know you're doing these — you can have your eyes open and do this breathing even as you're participating in other activities.

Instead of thinking about the upcoming test, try to use focus practices to bring your attention to your breath, body, or sounds.

Before the test starts, do RFI. Make sure you customize your RFI practice based on what worked best for you during practice exams.

After you set your intent, direct all your attention to your test — and test-take mindfully!

Test Day Obstacles

Distraction during the test

If you find yourself getting distracted with thoughts, sounds, or anything else during the test, gently bring yourself back to the test as soon as you've noticed your mind has wandered.

Don't be judgmental or unkind to yourself if this happens. It happens and it's totally normal, but now that you've trained in mindfulness, you have the skills to notice it and bring your mind back as soon as possible.

While you may be disappointed that you're distracted even after practicing meditation, you don't want to waste more time or energy scolding yourself. If thoughts like that come up, simply note that they're thoughts, and go back to your test.

Stress during the test

If you find yourself stressed out when you don't know an answer or have a difficult question during the test, take a deep breath. Then, use your preferred tool for dealing with distractions (Chapter 6). You may label the stress as a thought, name it as an emotion, or greet it as a visitor.

"Stress, I see that you're here. I can't engage with you right now, but I see you. I'll be back later."

After the naming, labeling, or greeting, direct your focus back to your test. Remember, test day is not the time to address and resolve any underlying stress in your life. The best you can do is acknowledge stress quickly and bring your focus back to your test.

Jitters

If you are literally shaking before your test, do a few belly breaths (Chapter 7).

If the jitters are still there and don't go away with some of the breathing techniques, then it's time to acknowledge them instead of trying to get rid of them:

Start by naming them. "There are these jitters I'm having."

Find them in your body. "My heart is racing; my stomach is fluttering."

Keep breathing as you notice these things.

Panic attack or freezing

No matter how much you practice and anticipate test anxiety, it's still possible to have a panic attack or freeze during an exam. If this happens, take a few deep breaths. Go back to the strategy you used to deal with text anxiety during practice exams. If you can't remember or didn't have time to practice beforehand, use this:

- Take a deep breath.
- Focus on your feet. Feel the hardness of the ground against your feet. What do your feet feel like right now? Can you feel the hard ground against you? Do your feet feel warm or cold? Do you feel any tingling sensations? Breathe as you bring your attention to your feet.
- When you can, gently bring your attention back to your test.

After the Test

You did it! Congratulations for completing your test. Don't abandon the mindfulness practices you've learned. They can also be helpful after the test.

Much of the stress related to tests comes from getting mad at yourself for making mistakes, anticipating your score, and the way you handle the score results after they come in.

There's nothing you can do about your test performance once it's over, so try not to think about the content of the test or how you did.

Try this to get your mind off of the outcome:

- One minute of relaxation practice (Chapter 7) to calm your nervous system.
- One minute of positive emotions practice (Chapter 8) — you deserve a little kindness and compassion after completing an important exam.

It's important to keep the momentum of your daily practice of mindfulness as well. Even if you are done with one test, you'll likely have another one soon.

Determining Your Next Steps

Once you get the test results, connect with your motivation for scoring well. Why were you studying? Why is scoring high important to you? Do your test results satisfy the reason you were aiming high for the test?

A mindful approach is not one of passivity. If you are not satisfied with your score, you may want to consider taking the test again, if that's an option — or studying harder for your next test. What mindfulness does do is allow you to make a clear decision on your next step, instead of blindly reacting.

Here's an example of spiraling thoughts that may accompany test results you're not satisfied with: "My score sucks. My life sucks. My future is ruined."

You can use your mindfulness practice to recognize that these are merely thoughts, and redirect your focus to an anchor. When you're able to calm your mind, you can make a rational decision on what your next step should be. That's a better outcome instead of making a knee-jerk emotional response or falling into a spiral of gloom and doom.

Realize It's Not the End of the World

When you get test results, it's natural to think your future happiness is tied to them. Yet, most events don't create lasting effects on happiness, no matter how important they may seem to be.

Researchers have found that events, such as passing or failing an exam, don't impact happiness as much as you may think they will. In fact, few experiences affect us for more than three months. As happiness researcher Daniel Gilbert states, "When good things happen, we celebrate for a while and then sober up. When bad things happen, we weep and whine for a while and then pick ourselves up and get on with it."[21]

Instead, it's the small things that you do every day that can add up to lasting happiness. Paying attention to the present moment and practicing gratitude have been shown to correlate with happiness.

If you're feeling bummed or sad about your test results, keep up with your mindfulness practices, especially your positive emotions practices. These will have a positive effect on your physical and mental health, regardless of the outcome of your test.

If you're happy with your results, take a moment to celebrate. Savor your happiness.

21 Daniel Gilbert. "The Science behind the Smile." Interview by Gardiner Morse. Harvard Business Review, January–February 2012, 84–8.

What You've Learned

Steps for success on test day:

✔ Take as many practice exams as possible to prepare yourself.

✔ Practice RFI and create a sequence that works best for you.

✔ Deal with stress and difficult emotions before the test so you don't get surprises on test day.

✔ Practice and be armed with tools for test anxiety.

✔ Be relaxed, calm, and focused during test day.

✔ Use mindfulness to face your test results with equanimity, realizing the effect on your happiness will be temporary.

✔ Keep building a mindfulness habit.

CONCLUSION

Congratulations for making it to the end of the book. You now see that staying focused on the present while you're taking a test is a worthwhile and achievable goal.

If you followed the steps in this book, you've been able to learn and practice a variety of mindfulness tools. Hopefully, you're already seeing positive effects in your test-taking — and your life.

I know some students prefer to read everything before trying out exercises. If that's you, that's okay. I hope that what you read has convinced you to give it a try.

As you practice studying and test-taking using mindfulness, you will find that you can be more present for other aspects of your life too: Your best friend telling you a story. The flowers in your garden. Even washing the dishes. When you immerse yourself in the present moment, life explodes with vibrancy and possibility.

Being present allowed you to find happiness in test-taking. So, too, will you find joy in those everyday places and mundane tasks, if you find yourself being more present.

Present moment awareness can sprinkle into your daily life and gradually transform it. It's hard to think of any part of life that isn't improved by being more fully present.

My hope is that mindfulness for test-taking will be just one step in a longer journey of self-discovery and reflection for you. I hope you'll find time to pause in moments of stillness, even as you march forward in the world achieving your goals.

Keep these three things in mind as you go forward with your journey:

1. **Make mindfulness your own path.** The steps in this book are guideposts. It's helpful to have a clear road map to begin with (which is why I wrote this book for you), but with practice, you'll adapt and customize the best mindfulness routines for yourself. Don't feel you're doing anything wrong if you veer from my instructions.

2. **You can do anything.** Learning mindfulness and applying it to boost your test-taking potential is impressive. You've learned how to focus your mind, establish a habit, and meet your goals. This skill set can help you be successful in any future endeavor. What will you do next?

3. **Know your purpose.** Keep in mind why you want to score well on tests. Beneath the surface of that goal, what are the values and priorities that are important to you? Keeping these in mind can help motivate you to keep achieving great things as well as put the outcome of your test in perspective.

I hope you reach your full potential with joy and happiness along the way.

ACKNOWLEDGMENTS

This book would not have been possible without the support and encouragement of my husband, Nishantha. Thank you for holding down the fort at home while I worked on this book and for providing me with frequent doses of good humor (and sometimes bad humor).

I owe a gigantic amount of thanks to my daughters, Shiyana and Ashani, who gave me the time I needed to write and who are my best cheerleaders. They were always ready to provide an opinion – and cuddles.

I'm so grateful to my parents, Ananda and Chinta Nimalasuriya, for their support and for always being there for me. I made a lot of progress on this book during trips to their house, nourished by delicious food.

I'm very thankful to the faculty at the Mindfulness Awareness Research Center at UCLA for the excellent training and teaching opportunities.

I'm immensely grateful for all my mindfulness teachers and students.

Special thanks to Cecilia, Jennifer, Kshamica, Lia, Rachel, and Yvonne for encouraging me and helping me get to the finishing line.

Thank you to Beacon Point LLC for insightful suggestions and editing.

ABOUT THE AUTHOR

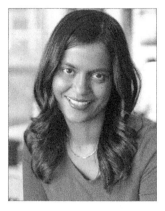

Nirosha Ruwan is a graduate of Harvard College and Harvard Law School, and she scored in the top one percent on the SAT and LSAT. She is a certified mindfulness teacher who coaches students of all ages on how to become high performers and reduce stress using mindfulness.

Because mindfulness has had such a positive impact on her life as a student and beyond, Nirosha is passionate about teaching mindfulness to others. She received her mindfulness facilitation training at the UCLA Mindfulness Awareness Research Center at the Semel Institute on Neuroscience and Human Behavior. Additionally, she is certified as a mindfulness teacher (Professional Level) by the International Mindfulness Teachers Association.

She hopes her readers discover a way to successfully take tests without succumbing to stress, overwhelm, and anxiety. If you'd like to find out Nirosha's latest offerings for students and test-takers, check out **www.MindOverScatterBook.com**

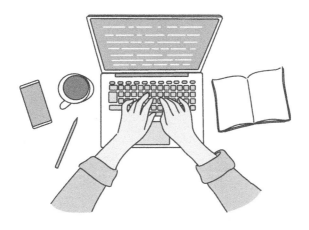

THANK YOU
FOR READING
MY BOOK!

I really appreciate all of your feedback,
and I love hearing what you have to say.
Please leave me a review on Amazon
letting me know what you thought
of the book.

Thanks so much!

Nirosha Ruwan

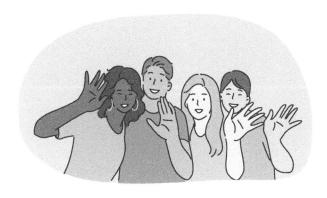

WHAT NEXT?

To get resources to help you implement
the steps in this book go to:

www.MindOverScatterBook.com

Made in the USA
Las Vegas, NV
25 February 2021

18565968R00089